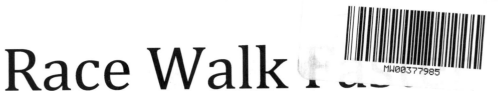

Race Walk Faster

by Training Smarter

An Intelligent Guide for Every Level Race Walker

by

Tim Seaman

Jeff Salvage

Copyright 2013, Walking Promotions

ISBN: 978-0-9827107-2-2

2nd Edition

Medford, NJ

Dedication

This book is dedicated to Stephan Plaetzer for his guidance and mentorship. His training philosophy was the basis for the concepts in the TEAMS training methodology.

This book is also dedicated to Diane Graham-Henry. Without her devotion to this project it would have never seen print.

Acknowledgements

We would like to thank Diane Graham-Henry for her tireless and repeated edits of this text as well as Stephan Plaetzer, Kjersti Plaetzer, Jaime Seaman, Tom Eastler, Maria Michta, Lauren Forgues, Rachel Seaman, Bruce Barron, Mike Shannon, Sabine Krantz, and Bastian Krantz for reviewing all or parts of this book.

In addition we would like to thank those coaches who influenced us over the years: Frank Manhardt, Mike DeWitt, Bohdan Bulakowski, Enrique Peña, Ray Khules, Gary Westerfield, Troy Engle, Frank Alongi, and Howard Jacobson.

Table of Contents

Chapter One - Introduction

Race Walk Faster by Training Smarter is for the countless coaches who say they do not know how to coach race walking, and for every athlete interested in training for our great event. Our previous texts, *Race Walk Clinic – in a Book* and *Race Walk like a Champion,* explain the techniques of race walking, and the latter text contains a general overview chapter on how to train. However, that chapter alone is not enough to completely develop a systematic training schedule suited to your specific situation. The needs of youth, high school, collegiate, elite, and masters athletes vary based on physiology and racing schedules, and one chapter cannot cover all of these intricacies.

Race Walk Faster by Training Smarter is an entire book devoted to training. We lay out the information required for a race walker to train at any level, and we assume no prior knowledge related to endurance training. The concepts are not hard to learn. Coaches of distance runners will find many of the concepts familiar – and not surprisingly, since race walking is an endurance event within the sport of track and field. The principles behind training a race walker are not much different from the principles behind training a distance runner for races of comparable length and time. Sure, race walkers take longer to complete the same distance, but concepts like periodization, proper recovery, and peaking all apply.

As with many topics, opinions on training philosophy vary widely. We recognize that there can be more than one path to the same result. Two different coaches may use two very different training philosophies and achieve similar success. So how do you decide whom to follow? We believe that how consistently a coach achieves results, especially in the most important events of his or her athletes' season, is the key factor in evaluating whether a training methodology has merit. Ultimately, every program is about peaking when it counts. Over the course of my career, I (Tim) have had the opportunity to work with some of the best coaches in America. These coaches produced Olympians; some of them produced Olympic medalists. While they all wanted the best for their athletes, the biggest problem I saw was the irregularity with which some of their athletes performed over the course of the season or from year to year.

As most coaches involved with race walking and track and field will tell you, the biggest problem they face is the consistency of their athletes. Some weeks they perform well, while at other times they seem off their game. Every coach's goal for his or her athletes is that they become stronger, faster, and more consistent as the season progresses. The question is how to do this.

Over my 20 years of race walking, I have significantly changed my training philosophy five times. My co-author Jeff Salvage has had similar experiences. We agree that the safest and most effective training program we know is based upon the teachings of Norwegian Coach Stephan Plaetzer. In the Team Plaetzer philosophy of endurance training, the main focus is one of balancing recovery and effort from the harder days. The program is not designed to get you in shape very quickly; instead, it is an adaptive system whereby athletes get stronger and stronger as the weeks and months go by, thus increasing their chances to peak when it counts. This approach contrasts with the styles of many coaches whose athletes walk their fastest race early in the season and then fade, usually due to overtraining. When that happens, the coach and athlete must ask themselves what they could have improved and what they could have changed. The answer is really simple. We call it the TEAMS (Tim's Elite Athlete Machine enhanced with Salvage) system of training.

Some will doubtlessly disagree with our philosophy. However, most athletes who have tried it find that it achieves better results with less stress than their previous methods.

Although *Race Walk Faster by Training Smarter* is designed to be a complete book on race walk training, it does not provide highly scientific explanations of physiological concepts. We believe that such discussions are too complicated to apply practically on a daily basis. Instead, *Race Walk Faster by Training Smarter* is a formula to help the masses train for race walking. It is a way for you to learn the TEAMS system so you can peak when it counts.

It is important to remember that no book can replace a knowledgeable high-level coach or advisor, either in developing a balanced, individualized training program or in providing feedback. Since there are relatively few experienced race walking coaches in the country (or the world), we've written *Race Walk Faster by Training Smarter* as a way to elevate your performance to a world class level.

Our training system provides more recovery time than many other training schedules. Many coaches push their athletes through a hard workout every other day, but the human body frequently needs more than just 48 hours to recover. Without a coach available to gauge how well you have recovered from the previous hard workout, you are likely to overtrain. Even with a coach watching, sometimes the athlete doesn't properly relay how tired he or she is. Jeff Salvage points out that, when he was coached from afar, he would often enthusiastically call his coach after the good workouts, but not always after the bad ones. This practice could have led his coach to think he was recovering from the harder workouts better than he was. Don't let this happen to you.

Our training plan also offers you more flexibility should you need an extra day of rest because you had to rush the kids to soccer practice or study for an exam and are too fatigued to train. We believe this greater flexibility helps you succeed both in race walking and in life.

The most efficient way to get better, faster, and stronger is to be consistent in your training. If you have some great days and some horrible days, you are teaching your body and mind to be inconsistent. In previous training programs I have had a few "gold medal" weeks of training when every single workout was as fast as it could possibly be. At the end of those weeks I would say to myself, "Holy cow, how did I do that?" Unfortunately the gold medal week was of no value if it left me too tired to perform at my best in competition. With the TEAMS training philosophy you will not have those gold medal training weeks; instead you are going to have many "silver medal" weeks (with solid training but without all-out exertion and exhaustion) stacked together over a longer period of time. The continual buildup of this strong training is best suited to produce the gold medal when you really want it, at the peak of your season.

In this book we first explain the essential components of the TEAMS training program and then show you how to build them into a sensible, complete program. As assembling the parts may still seem difficult for some readers, we provide sample schedules for race walkers at all levels. We recognize that the needs of youth race walkers differ from those of elite or masters walkers. Competitors at different levels not only race different distances, but may race with dramatically different frequency. Younger walkers often recover more quickly than their more mature counterparts. For this reason, we have developed specific schedules for five groups: youth, high school, collegiate, aspiring elite, and masters athletes. Since even these categories of race walkers are broad, we further break down some of them into smaller groups with schedules defined to their specific requirements.

Some of the training philosophies I have used in the past made me so tired that I wanted to sleep twelve hours a day. Every workout felt like a race. At the end of each session I felt as if I could not go another step at that pace. I never felt this way when training with my Team Plaetzer teammates, and you don't need to feel this way either. With the TEAMS system you will almost always feel as if you could keep going, or go faster, if you were asked to do so. The benefit of this type of training is that you can walk more miles, feel stronger, and be ready to fight when the time comes for that peak race. Many of the athletes using this type of training constantly tell me they are amazed at how easy the training is and how well they are performing without killing themselves.

We often say that the TEAMS approach first builds the engine and then fine-tunes it to perform at its peak when it counts most. You can't put your foot on the accelerator if you just have two cylinders. Your "car" will not go anywhere fast. You must build the engine in its entirety before going to the racetrack. In 2004, Kevin Eastler and I built our engines in this way and achieved the best race walk finishes by Americans at the Olympic Games in 24 years. We also had the two all-time fastest American race walking performances in the Olympic Games ever. When we put the pedal to the floor we passed and beat two Russians, two Chinese, and two Mexicans—six Olympic athletes from three of the best race walking countries in the world.

How was this possible? Through consistency of training, team work, and surrounding ourselves with positive people, we performed better internationally then we had before. Thus far, this system of training, and the Team Plaetzer system it's based upon, has produced two Olympic silver medals and four U.S. Olympic Team spots, as well as the U.S. 30km, 20km, 15km, and 10km road records and the 5,000m indoor record. It also brought Norway's Erik Tysse, "The Rocket," to world-class status, including a fifth-place finish in the 50km walk at the 2008 Beijing Olympics. It has taken a 16-year-old American male who was willing to follow the program diligently to National Junior records at 5, 10, and 20 kilometers as well as a 4th-place finish at the World Youth Track and Field Championships in just under a year.

Do you want to maximize your own success? Are you ready to be added to the list of athletes succeeding with TEAMS? If so, then let's turn the page and begin.

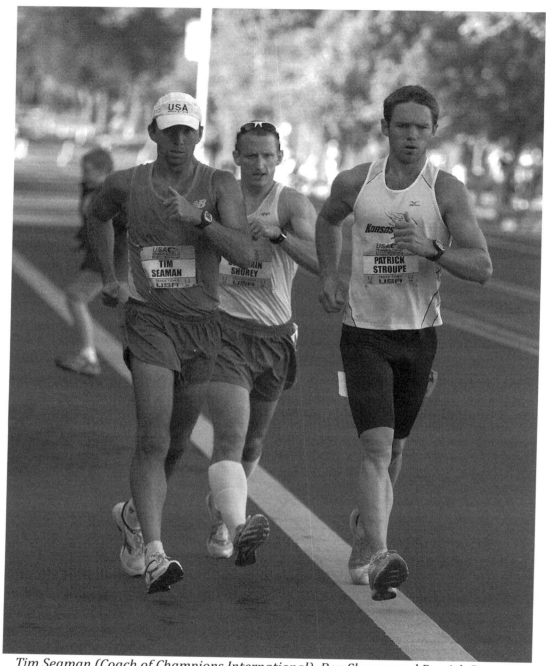

Tim Seaman (Coach of Champions International), Ben Shorey, and Patrick Stroupe in the lead pack at the 2009 20km Nationals

Chapter Two: Building a Training Program

Before you can actually construct a training schedule, you must understand each of the individual pieces of the puzzle. In this chapter, we explain all the key components in building a training program. Then, in the next chapter we show how to assemble a season-long training schedule.

Most coaches agree that walking the exact same distance at the exact same pace seven days a week isn't a path to success. Instead, modern training programs vary workouts in distance and intensity. These workouts are called by many names, but are often variations of the same basic components. In *Race Walk Faster by Training Smarter* we break them into three broad categories of workouts. They are the Endurance Zone workouts (or Zone #1), Speed Endurance workouts (Zone #2 or Zone #3 – depending on how far along you are in the season), and Speed Repeats (Zone #3 or Zone #4 – depending on how far along you are in the season and the distance of each repeat). In addition, one can also perform tempo and progression walks, although these are used sparingly in the TEAMS system. The bulk of the workouts are in Zone #1, with each progressively harder zone comprising less and less of the volume of training. This is illustrated in the following training pyramid figure:

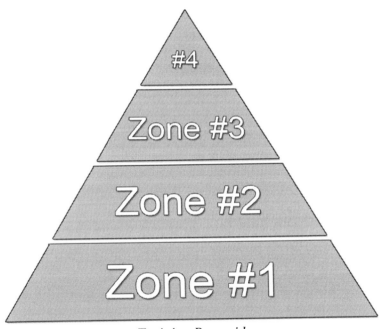

Training Pyramid

Just walking is not enough. Great race walking technique is not acquired solely by focusing on how to walk. Instead, a walker must perform range of motion drills that we call technique drills, cool down stretches, as well as strength training exercises. These drills, stretches, and exercises are explained in detail in *Race Walk Clinic in a Book* and are merely referenced and prescribed in this text.

11

Definition of the Zones

The TEAMS philosophy is based on workouts that vary in level of effort. The four workout zones correspond to increasingly difficult walking intensities. The challenge for many is to determine the proper walking intensity for each zone. Since the intensity of each workout in TEAMS is denoted by a zone number, it is important to explain how to determine what your walking intensity should be for Zone #1, #2, #3 and #4 workouts.

There are three methods to determine how fast you should walk your workouts in each zone:

- Heart rate based
- Race/Speed pace based
- Lactate test based

Heart Rate as Basis for Workout Pace

The most traditional way to determine your race walking pace in each zone is to base it on your heart rate. Our definition of the zones may differ slightly from others, so if you are comparing TEAMS to another system, make sure the terms being compared are compatible.

In heart rate based determination, each zone has a corresponding heart rate range that the athlete should maintain while walking. This range is expressed in percentage of your theoretical maximum heart rate. See Table 2-1 for the ranges used for Zone #1 to Zone #4 workouts.

Zone	% of Theoretical Max Heart Rate
#1	70% - 75%
#2	76% - 85%
#3	86% - 90%
#4	91% - 95%

Table 2-1

In order to use this method you must know your theoretical maximum heart rate. You can determine it by pushing yourself to the maximum in a hard workout or race, or you can use a formula to estimate it.

If you want to try to reach your theoretical maximum in a workout, try warming up really well for about two or three kilometers. Perform your normal warm-up drills and any stretches you may consider pertinent. Now, walk 400 meters at your one-mile race pace. Rest for 30 seconds and then blast through a 200-meter interval at full speed. Immediately after the 200-meter sprint, obtain your heart rate, either from a heart rate monitor or by counting your pulse for 10 seconds and multiplying by 6. Rest for 2 minutes, including the time it takes to obtain your heart rate, then repeat the effort (400 meters fast, 30 seconds of rest, and 200-meter sprint). Again obtain your heart rate at the beginning of a two minute rest period. Repeat this sequence, until your heart rate stops increasing. Probably no more than four or five sets are required, though this number can vary. The highest value obtained should be a close approximation of your maximum.

There are many reasons why you may not be able to achieve your theoretical maximum heart rate while race walking. New walkers still working on their technique or muscle strength will not reach maximum heart rate, nor will walkers who have also trained significantly more in other highly aerobic activities. If you use the highest heart rate recorded in a race as your maximum, ask yourself if you could have pushed a little harder for a short spurt. If so, then you can probably add a few beats to your highest heart rate recorded during the race and call that your theoretical maximum.

I reached a maximum of 195 at the 2004 Indoor Nationals 5km walk. As John Nunn and I battled for the win, I walked the last kilometer in 3:43 and finished completely exhausted. I could not have pushed any faster at any point in time during those last few laps. So I could confidently call 195 my theoretical maximum, Interestingly, John Nunn also achieved his highest recorded heart rate that day—205! That is the sign of an athlete at peak fitness and one who knows how to race, and a testament to the battle that we waged that day.

So if my theoretical maximum heart rate is 195, my Zone #1 heart rate should be between 70 and 75 percent of 195, or about 137 to 146 beats per minute. Similarly, rates for Zones #2 through #4 can be calculated as we have done for myself in Table 2-2.

Tim's Zone #	Tim's Heart Rate Range
#1	137 – 146
#2	148 – 166
#3	168 – 176
#4	177 – 185

Table 2-2

If you cannot obtain your maximum heart rate directly, you can use the estimation tool described by Jeff Salvage in *Race Walk like a Champion*:

(220 - Age - Resting Heart Rate[1]) * Percent Maximum Heart Rate + Resting Heart Rate

---

[1] Resting heart rate is calculated by taking your heart rate when you first awaken in the morning and are still in bed. Take your heart rate for 10 seconds and multiple the number by 6.

By way of illustration, if I used this formula to estimate my desired Zone #1 heart rate, I would use my age (37), my resting heart rate (40), and the range of 70 to 75 percent of my maximum heart rate. I could thus calculate the lower end of my Zone #1 training heart rate as:

$$(220 - 37 - 40) * .70 + 40 = 140.1$$

And the upper end of my Zone #1 training heart rate would be:

$$(220 - 37 - 40) * .75 + 40 = 147.25$$

The result is reasonably close to the numbers (137 to 146) that I obtained when using my directly obtained maximum heart rate. Table 2-3 summarizes my heart rate zones for both physical and formula-based calculations.

Tim's Zone #	Tim's Physical Heart Rate Zone	Tim's Formula Based Zones
#1	137 – 146	140 - 147
#2	148 – 166	149-162
#3	168 – 176	163-169
#4	177 – 185	170-176

Table 2-3

As you become comfortable with training in zones, you will begin to know what pace is normally associated with your desired heart rate range. However, do not rely solely on your pace when you train, as many factors could affect your pace on a given day. Warmer temperatures can cause you to sweat faster, become more dehydrated, and walk more slowly than you normally do at a given heart rate. Similarly, training at altitude will slow you down by approximately three percent of your normal speed for each mile of altitude. Additionally, stress, lack of sleep, or the onset of an illness can also alter your heart rate. When your engine speaks up, don't ignore it. Listen to your body and adjust your pace to match the proper Zone #1 heart rate so as not to risk overtraining.

So remember, your heart rate monitor is the best training partner you will ever have. Make sure you listen to it. If you are serious about race walking, you really should purchase a heart rate monitor. It is the principal tool used in this training program and will be your most valuable training partner.

Note that not all walkers can use heart rate as their guide. Some masters athletes may be on beta blockers or other medication that effects their heart rate. If you have a specific medical condition, please consult your doctor for advice.

Race Pace as Basis for Workout Pace

For some, heart rate monitors might be cumbersome, cost too much, or just not work consistently. In these cases there is a second, albeit slightly less accurate, way to figure out your appropriate pace for your workouts in each zone. If you have raced at 10 or 20 kilometers, you can use a percentage of the per-kilometer pace of your best recent time. "Recent" is subjective and depends upon what has happened in your life since your best performance. If no major changes have occurred, and you are still very fit, you can use your best time in the last year. However, if you walked your best time once two years ago and then never came close again, you should use a race pace that is consistent with a more recent performance.

The calculation is straightforward, but certainly not quick. If you wish, follow the math and perform the calculations yourself. If you do not wish to perform the calculations yourself, please see the chart in Appendix C to look up your appropriate training pace in each zone. Using the TEAMS system, athletes should walk their zone workouts as a percentage of their 20km (or 10km) race pace as shown in Table 2-4:

TEAMS' Zone #	% of 20km Race Pace	% of 10km Race Pace
#1	77% to 84%	72% to 80%
#2	85% - 94%	81% to 89%
#3	95% - 105%	90% to 100%
#4	106% - 110%	101% -

Table 2-4

If you have properly trained for and raced a 20km, it is preferable to use the 20km values. The 10km values are provided only as an estimate for walkers who have not yet competed at 20km.

Taking Zone #1 workouts as our illustration, the easiest way to calculate a desired race pace is to find your 20km pace per kilometer and then multiply by 1/.84 and 1/.77 to find the slow and fast extremes, respectively, of my range. You could also calculate your speed in meters per second, multiply by .770 and .840, and then convert back to time per kilometer, but that is much more complicated.

For example, while my personal best time for 20km is 1:22:02, I am not likely to consistently walk that time again. A time such as 1:23:20 or 4:10/km is a more pragmatic estimation of my current 20km potential. I convert 4:10 to 250 seconds, multiply by 1/.84 and 1/.77, and get 298 and 325 seconds, which means a training pace of 4:58 to 5:25 per kilometer.

My actual Zone #1 pace as determined by my heart rate is 5:05 to 5:20 per kilometer, so using my race pace is a reasonable though not perfect estimation. This is shown in Table 2-5.

TEAMS' Zone #	% 20 km Race Pace	Tim's Pace Range
#1	77% - 84%	5:25/km – 4:58/km
#2	85% - 94%	4:54/km - 4:26/km
#3	95% - 105%	4:23/km – 3:58/km
#4	106% - 110%	3:55/km - 3:47/km

Table 2-5

Lactate as Basis for Workout Pace

A third method to determine your proper training pace is to measure the amount of blood lactate at various paces while race walking. While you are working out your muscles produce blood lactate, a byproduct of a lack of oxygen in the blood. At slow walking intensities the levels of production and removal of blood lactate in your body are equal and thus it remains stable in your system. However, at faster walking paces, the amount of lactate produced exceeds the amount that your body can clear from its system. Eventually, this lactate buildup forces the athlete to slow down. As one gets in better shape, one can walk at faster paces for longer durations while producing less blood lactate. By measuring your level of blood lactate, you can see how the muscles are working at a given pace and customize your training program accordingly.

Blood lactate is measured in millimoles per liter of blood (mmol/L). In Table 2-6, each zone workout has a corresponding level of millimoles per liter for the desired blood lactate level. For example, Zone #1 workouts should have blood lactate at or under 1.2 millimoles per liter.

TEAMS' Zone #	mmol/L
#1	< 1.2
#2	2.0 – 3.4
#3	3.5 – 4.4
#4	>= 4.5

Table 2-6

An issue with lactate testing is that the machines used for this purpose are not cheap. The machine we used, the Lactate Pro, is a great help to our training, but it costs over $400. Serious athletes will want to purchase one; for beginners, the heart rate monitor is a smarter first investment.

With a lactate machine, a small amount of blood is taken and placed onto a lactate strip (each strip costs about $2). Within 60 seconds the machine indicates how much lactate is in your blood. Most protocols require that you take multiple samples to determine your blood lactate at different paces.

16

By taking more than one sample, you can draw a blood lactate curve from the sampled points and extrapolate the estimated blood lactate levels for any training pace.

You must calibrate the machine with each individual box of lactate strips that you receive, or the results will not be accurate. Also, it is extremely important to make sure that only the drop of blood, not your finger, touches the strip, because the sweat on your finger will cause an erroneous result.

The protocol that we follow for developing a blood lactate curve requires a walker to repeat a number of intervals at a varied pace with a steady, prescribed progression. We have our more experienced walkers complete six or seven intervals of two kilometers each, with about two minutes rest in between each one (including the time needed for the test). Determining the pace for the first interval may involve a little trial and error, but the intention is to start slightly slower than Zone #1 pace and then walk 1/2 kilometer per hour faster than the previous interval each time. See Appendix A for assistance with pacing. The first few intervals should feel ridiculously easy, and the last interval should be slightly faster than your 10km or 20km race pace. Don't rush and pick a faster starting pace, because the early readings are important in developing an accurate blood lactate curve; without them you will not be able to determine a Zone #1 pace. Later samples are used to determine your lactate threshold. Please note that this protocol is too advanced for youth athletes unless they are already walking at an elite level. Instead, try a shorter interval like 1200m or 1600m. Please note, in the following chapters when a training schedule prescribes "Lactate Test," these protocols should be used for the day's workout.

Figure 2-1 shows the results of a recent lactate test. The graph shows the non linear progression of blood lactate levels. This is fairly common, but it is sometimes depicted by showing an inaccurate representation as a smooth curve. My Zone #1 blood lactate level of 1.2 millimoles/liter (mmol/L) and my lactate threshold are highlighted with vertical lines in the figure.

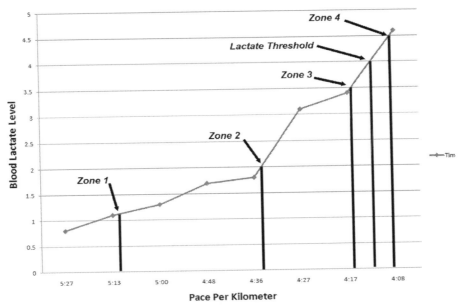

Figure 2-1

The numbers on the vertical axis of the graph represent the millimoles per liter of lactate (mmol/L); and the numbers on the horizontal axis represent pace per kilometer. A properly executed protocol shows a steady increase in speed as well as an increased production of lactate. As more lactate is produced, the muscles become more and more fatigued. Eventually you reach a point where the body cannot "clear" the lactate and the body cannot continue. Exhaustion sets in and you slow down. Some well trained athletes vary from this lactate progression, their training enables them to be more efficient at certain faster speeds.

The paces indicated by my lactate tests come very close to the zone times derived from the other methods. For example, the pace-based method set my Zone #1 training pace at 4:58 to 5:25 per kilometer; I reached 1.2 mmol/L of lactate at 5:13 per kilometer. This test was performed early in a training season; as the season progresses and my condition improves, the vertical line marking my pace at 1.2 mmol/L should shift to the right (i.e., aligning with a faster training pace). If it does, that means I am producing less lactate at a given pace and I am capable of walking faster with the same amount of effort.

The lactate test is also a great way of estimating about how fast you should be able to walk for a given distance. For example, a well-trained race walker can typically hold a lactate level of 1.5 to 2.0 mmol/L for a 50km race, 2.5 to 3.0 mmol/L for 30km, or 3.5 to 4.5 mmol/L for 20km. We have also found that an elite race walker can hold around 5 mmol/L for 10 kilometers and 6 mmol/L or higher for 5 kilometers.

Race Distance	mmol/L
5km	6 +
10km	5
20km	3.5 to 4.5
30km	2.5 to 3.0
50km	1.5 to 2

Table 2-7

Most athletes, if they try to walk an entire 20km race while producing over 4 mmol/L of lactate, will crash during the last few kilometers. I recommend that you walk at a speed that will keep your lactate just under 4.0 mmol/L for as long as possible so that your body can clear the lactate and you can continue to walk at a fast speed. You should be able to start your "kick" and thus pop over 4 mmol/L with a few kilometers to go if you have followed your training plan properly and finish strong instead of crawling to the finish.

Endurance Zone Workouts – Zone #1

The endurance zone workouts, also called Zone #1, are the largest component of TEAMS training. They are the backbone for recovering from the harder days and are used to build the foundation of the engine. In a nutshell, they are easy-paced workouts that:

- Become the base work, or foundation, of our training schedule
- Burn fat
- Build your engine
- Aid consistency of training
- Aid recovery from the harder sessions

Almost all training programs have some form of Zone #1 workouts; they may be known as easy days, recovery days, or long slow distance. The key in TEAMS is to make sure that your Zone #1 workouts are performed at the proper pace. Unfortunately, before I adopted this training approach, I used to walk my recovery days a mere 10-15 seconds slower per kilometer (15-25 seconds per mile) than my 20km personal record (PR). As crazy as that sounds, I did it for five utterly exhausting years. Thankfully, four-time Olympic gold medalist Robert Korzeniowski and Stephan Plaetzer set me straight in 2003. Korzeniowski looked at my plan and told me there was no way he could follow it and peak properly. At the time, I was following instructions to walk between 4:20 and 4:25 per kilometer (7:00 to 7:10 per mile) on my easy days. Korzeniowski indicated his easy days were at 4:50/km (7:45/mile) and it was crazy for me to walk almost 30 seconds faster per kilometer than he was walking. To put it in perspective, at the time my PR for the 20km was about four minutes slower than his. In fact, my recovery-day walking pace was close to 95 percent of my race pace! No wonder I would be strong for the first race of each season but then get progressively weaker as the season wore on.

It took a while for me to grasp and accept their explanation, but gradually I became a believer. Belief turned into success and, after years of trying, I was finally able to break the U.S. 20km record with a time of 1:22:02. I was able to accomplish this lifelong goal by walking slower on my easy days. You too can accomplish your goals if you follow this training system with dedication, discipline, and a positive mental outlook.

Walking the Zone #1 workouts at too high a heart rate does not allow proper recovery. Your Zone #1 workouts will seem too slow at first; be patient, because as you progress your times will come down. The added consistency of training builds your engine bigger and stronger, with immensely improved results and a greater chance of peaking when it counts.

After my breakthrough 2004 season I analyzed my training logs from 2003 and 2004. I found that in 2003 I had walked faster than 5 minutes per kilometer 83 times on days that were categorized as easy! Those 83 days did not even include the faster efforts (speedwork sessions, fartlek sessions, and races). They were supposed to be recovery days. In contrast, in 2004 I had only three days when I finished a Zone #1 workout at faster than a five minute per kilometer pace. Both years had about the same number of speedwork or fartlek sessions, but the difference was I had 80 more days of recovery from those harder sessions in 2004 than in 2003. Instead of feeling as if I had just completed a race every few days, my body was able to adapt and absorb the harder days, and the end result was that I was able to walk more consistently and faster.

Before Trevor Barron, 2009 Junior National Champion, started training with me under this system his best time for 10km was over 50 minutes. Within five months of training he lowered his time to 46:18, at the IAAF World Race Walking Cup in Russia in May 2008. After a five-month break to run for his high school cross country team, he resumed race walking in November 2008. In July 2009 he walked 10 kilometers in 42:22, breaking the U.S. Junior Record and placing fourth in the World Youth Championships. He made this improvement while walking two hard workouts per week. Ask him how he was able to have such a great season and he will say that strictly observing his proper Zone #1 pace had a lot to do with it. Trevor is a believer, and you should be as well.

TALES FROM THE TRACK

In 2009 we reconfirmed this system with a willing, diligent junior athlete, Trevor Barron, then age 16. According to our testing of Trevor, we knew that at a given heart rate we could expect his lactate to be at a certain level. For example, we knew that at a heart rate of 192-194, Trevor's lactate was right around 5.0 mmol/L, but if his heart rate went up to 196 his lactate would jump to nearly 6.0 mmol/L and he would be unable to maintain his pace for very long.

Athletes can't check their lactate during a race, but they can wear a heart rate monitor. We analyzed Trevor's monitor readings after the U.S. Junior Nationals, where he won comfortably, but pushed himself hard for the last 5km; and the World Youth (under-17) Championships in Italy where he worked his way from 20th to 3rd place. He held 3rd place for a brief moment and then slipped back to 4th. We noticed in both 10km races he could not maintain his heart rate above 194 for very long and, in fact, began to slow down shortly after his heart rate reached 195. Physiologically, at this point he was accumulating significantly more lactate than his body could remove or clear from his muscles. Trevor applied this information in his final race of 2009, the Pan-American Junior Track and Field Championships. As a result he was able to speed up in the last two kilometers without crashing while other athletes wilted in the heat, finishing a close fourth as the youngest athlete in a 19-and-under race.

Speed Endurance/Fartlek Workouts

The second type of workouts in the TEAMS arsenal are called Speed Endurance. These are fartleks whereby you alternate between "fast" and "slow" walking. The fast parts are done in either Zone #2 or Zone #3, depending on the distance. The slower portions of the workout are walked in Zone #1.

From 1998 to 2007, while winning 10 consecutive Indoor Championships 5,000 meter titles, I was trained by three different coaches with three different philosophies. The first two training regiments would push my body to the limits of utter exhaustion three times a week with speed repeat workouts. Both coaches said I had the talent to break Tim Lewis's American record time of 19:18. Both coaches said I had the mental fortitude and physical resilience to withstand the training necessary to do it. The systems made me very fast for short distances, but neither of them could give me the speed endurance capacity required to maintain a record pace for five kilometers. In 2006, after using the Team Plaetzer method of training, I was finally able to cut my time to 19:15.88 and break Tim Lewis' 19-year-old American Record.

What had changed? Before 2003, I used fartleks (workouts with fast and slow components intermixed throughout the workout without stopping race walking at any point) as a secondary workout to speed repeats (fast intervals repeated with significant rest between intervals). In contrast, after 2003, Coach Plaetzer applied Robert Korzeniowski's preference for fartleks over speed repeats. As Korzeniowski put it, you don't get to stop in the middle of a race, so why train like that? Fartleks enabled Korzeniowski's body to adapt more quickly to walking long distances and helped him to walk his way to four Olympic gold medals.

Speed endurance workouts fine tune your engine so that it performs better and more efficiently on race day. Speed endurance workouts differ from traditional speed workouts in that they work both the speed component and the endurance component at the same time. This contrasts with my earlier interval workouts that focused primarily on walking at top speed. Programs that focus too much on walking at top speed of a walker are developing a pace that nobody can use in a distance race. Salvage had a similar philosophy when developing his training schedules for *Race Walk Like a Champion*. Instead of training faster than race pace for the majority of faster paced walking, Salvage prescribed walking at or slightly slower than race pace for most of your speed intervals. However, in the *Race Walk Like a Champion* schedules, the majority of speedwork consisted of variations of walking at a fast pace, resting for a short break to recover, and then walking fast again. This is called interval training. In contrast, Korzeniowski walked the majority of his fast paced training as fartlek sessions.

Speed endurance workouts are also great for youngsters or for athletes new to race walking. At the Junior Olympic level, almost invariably one or more inexperienced walkers start out at a sprint and eventually crash, finishing off the medal podium. The young walker's adrenaline is pumping and, without the proper training and coaching, he or she falls victim to the excitement. By properly training with speed endurance, the same walker can become familiar with the correct starting pace. As a race goes on and improperly trained walkers start to fade, the base of speed endurance allows properly trained walkers to continue at or accelerate their pace. I instill in my athletes that the first kilometer (or the first 200 meters for youths) should always be the slowest. It should never be, as is often the case, the fastest. Walkers who sprint off the start line will spike their lactate and make their legs feel like lead bricks. When it comes down to the final sprint, almost always the person who started fastest will lose to someone who started smarter and didn't push hard from the beginning.

Examples of Speed Endurance/Fartlek Workouts

There are many ways to vary speed endurance or fartlek workouts. Stronger, more experienced walkers will include more intervals in their sessions, while beginners and younger walkers will have fewer intervals. As with any training, you must remember to not do too much too soon. Don't be a weekend warrior. If you haven't walked the 1km/500m fartlek before, even if you are an advanced athlete don't start with 14 sets the first time; rather, increase the number later in the season as you progressively get stronger. Here are some sample workouts.

Speed Distance: 500m	Heart Rate Based Pace: Zone #3 Speed Based Pace: Zone #3 Lactate Based Pace: up to 4.5 mmol/L	Level: Beginner to advanced
Easy Distance: 500m	Easy Pace: Zone #1	# of Intervals: 4 - 20
Notes: Your heart rate should drop at least 10 to 15 percent during the easy distance portions. This is a great workout for resuming speed endurance training a few days after a hard race. Two-time U.S. Olympic walker Allen James coined the title "Special K" for this workout because Robert Korzeniowski frequently used a similar workout pattern.		

Speed Distance: 800m	Heart Rate Based Pace: Zone #3 Speed Based Pace: Zone #3 Lactate Based Pace: up to 4.5 mmol/L	Level: Beginner to Advanced
Easy Distance: 400m	Easy Pace: Zone #1	# of Intervals: 3 - 12
Notes: Known as the Spanish Fartlek, this combination is used frequently in the Spanish system of training as a way to keep walkers' leg speed up during their high mileage weeks.		

Speed Distance: 1 km	Heart Rate Based Pace: Zone #3 Speed Based Pace: Zone #3 Lactate Based Pace: 3.0 to 4.5 mmol/L	Level: Moderate to Advanced
Easy Distance: 500 m	Easy Pace: Zone #1	# of Intervals: 5 - 14
Notes: Solid workout that works on both your speed and your speed endurance, especially for those athletes wanting to excel at distances above 10km and above.		

Speed Distance: 2km	Heart Rate Based Pace: Zone #3 Speed Based Pace: Zone #3 Lactate Based Pace: 3.0 to 4.5 mmol/L	Level: Moderate to Advanced
Easy Distance: 1km	Easy Pace: Zone #1	# of Intervals: 4 to 7
Notes: Very tough workout. Advanced athletes should do these intervals at their 20km race pace; younger or less experienced athletes can do them around their 10km race pace.		

Speed Distance: 4km	Heart Rate Based Pace: Zone #2 or #3 Speed Based Pace: Zone #2 or #3 Lactate Based Pace: 3.0 to 4.0 mmol/L	Level: Advanced
Easy Distance: 1km	Easy Pace: Zone #1	# of Intervals: 2 to 4
Notes: This workout really builds your engine and contributes to 20km training, but it is only for those who are training at a high level.		

Speed Distance: 5km	Heart Rate Based Pace: Zone #2 or #3 Speed Based Pace: 20km race pace Lactate Based Pace: 2.0 to 4.0 mmol/L	Level: Advanced
Easy Distance: 1km	Easy Pace: Zone #1	# of Intervals: 2 or 3
Notes: Another very hard workout, usually done just under your 20km pace. Slightly slower will still be useful, but going too fast will risk wearing you out in training.		

Bohdan's Rhythm

Named after Polish walker Bohdan Bulakowski, who placed seventh in the 20km walk at the 1980 Moscow Olympics, this fartlek is not to be taken lightly. Bulakowski coached U.S. walkers prior to the 1996 Atlanta Olympics and also at the U.S. Olympic Training Center in Chula Vista, CA. He emphasized "professionalism," especially staying fully focused during training, to his athletes. Focus was especially important during this workout because of the many speed changes involved, but this is a great workout to prepare for a short race and a wonderful introduction to fartlek training for youths and beginner walkers. It permits you to focus on technique while walking fast for short distances.

First, warm up well for two or three kilometers and do some mobility and technique drills. Next, walk 100m hard followed immediately by 100 meters easy. Once you complete the easy 100m, then walk 200m hard, again followed immediately by 100 meters easy. This is then followed with 300m hard, 100 easy, 400m hard and 100m easy. This is shown in Figure 2-2.

Figure 2-2

Speed Distance: 100, 200, 300, 400m	Heart Rate Based Pace: Zone #4 Speed Based Pace: Zone #4 Lactate Based Pace: > 4.5 mmol/L	Level: Beginner to advanced
Easy Distance: 100m	Easy Pace: Zone #1	# of Intervals: 2 to 4
Notes: Repeat this sequence 2 to 4 times but don't stop between sets; just walk 100m easy and then begin again.		

Within each set you should keep the same pace in each hard effort, and as you move into a new set your pace should stay the same or get faster. The faster portions of this workout are done in Zone #4 and the slower parts are done in Zone #1. The workout may seem easy due to the relatively short fast bursts, but if you walk it in Zone #4 it is not. As one of my athletes just told me recently after doing it for the first time, "Holy cow, it really kicked my butt!"

This workout is especially good for beginners and masters walkers who have problems with too much double contact (i.e., having both feet on the ground for too long). It allows them to feel what it is like to extend their stride length and range of motion to the verge of lifting (i.e., having both feet off the ground for a brief instant). Typically the speeds reached will be useful only for very short

23

distance races such as a mile or 3,000 meters. However, it will help you clear the rust from your engine when you haven't gone fast in a while and can be a fun workout for the kids.

Remember, don't burn yourself out in these workouts. Athletes who consistently push their bodies over 90 percent of their maximum heart rate, faster than their 20km race pace, or well over 4 mmol/L in their training have a high probability of burning out halfway through the season or getting injured. Restrain your effort so as not to push the body too hard. The goal of a training session should be to train, not to race! Racing in a training workout depletes your reserves and results in overtraining and declining performance.

Time Based Fartleks:
If you don't have a measured course nearby, you can still do fartleks—just measure time instead of distance. Here are three possibilities.

Norwegian Fartlek
Fellow Olympian Kevin Eastler once said this is "the hardest workout that I ever did in my life."

Speed Time: 2,4,6,8,7,5,3,1 minutes	**Heart Rate Based Pace:** Zone #3 **Speed Based Pace:** Zone #3	**Level:** Moderate to Advanced
Active Recovery Time: 2 min	**Lactate Based Pace:** up to 4.5 mmol/L	**# of Intervals:** 1
Notes: This is a 50-minute fartlek whereby you walk pickups of 2,4,6,8,7,5,3,1 minutes with 2 min of Zone #1 walking between. The pickups are done at your Zone #3 heart rate or the corresponding pace and lactate. The first two pickups will feel short and easy; as they get longer, be careful not to push too hard.		

Elite walkers doing this workout will check for their 10km split, assuming that they reach it. If you don't have a measured course, try to walk in one direction for 25 minutes and then turnaround, remembering where you turned around until the next time you do this workout to see if you are getting faster.

Kevin's Fartlek
Named after Kevin Eastler, this fartlek contains equal periods of fast walking and recovery walking. The pickup lengths, in minutes, are 1, 2, 3, 4, 5, 4, 3, 2, 1 minutes. Thus you would walk one minute fast (Zone #3) and one easy (Zone #1), two minutes fast and two minutes easy, and so forth.

Speed Time: 1,2,3,4,5,4,3,2,1 minutes	**Heart Rate Based Pace:** Zone #3 **Speed Based Pace:** Zone #3	**Level:** Moderate to Advanced
Active Recovery Time: Equal rest	**Lactate Based Pace:** up to 4.5 mmol/L	# of Intervals: 1
Notes: This is a 50- minute fartlek whereby you do pickups of 1,2,3,4,5,4,3,2,1 minutes with equal rest of Zone #1 walking between. The pickups are done at your Zone #3 heart rate or the corresponding pace and lactate. The first two pickups will feel short and easy; as they get longer, be careful not to push too hard.		

Super Norwegian Fartlek

This workout is a favorite of Erik Tysse and one that you should not undertake unless you are well trained.

Speed Time: 2,4,6,8,10,9,7,5,3,1 minutes	Heart Rate Based Pace: Zone #3 Speed Based Pace: Zone #3	Level: Advanced
Active Recovery Time: 2 min	Lactate Based Pace: up to 4.5 mmol/L	# of Intervals: 1
Notes: This is a 73-minute fartlek whereby you walk pickups of 2,4,6,8,10,9,7,5,3,1 minutes with 2 min of Zone #1 walking between. The pickups are done at your Zone #3 heart rate or the corresponding pace and lactate. The first two pickups will feel short and easy; as they get longer, be careful not to push too hard.		

Speed Repeats

The TEAMS system of training also uses speed repeat workouts, but very sparingly. These are generally Zone #3 or Zone #4 workouts, depending on the distances walked. In the later part of base training, speed repeats can be used if fartleks still feel too difficult, but in this case they should function as a transition to fartleks and shouldn't be continued very long. The other time when speed repeats are used is during the Peak phase of training.

After you have performed a few months of fartleks, speed repeats feel easier in comparison. You might wonder why you are taking a break in the middle of the workout when you feel as if you could just keep walking, but the breaks allow your body to push hard without unduly stressing it. They prepare you to peak for the big race that is just around the corner.

Speed repeat sessions are like fartleks, but instead of walking easy in between hard efforts, you completely stop. Sometimes, while you rest, you may do a few stretches, but the idea is to partially recover aerobically from the effort of the fast-paced interval. The key to speed repeat sessions is to avoid taking too long, or too short, a break and thus allowing your heart rate not to drop too low, or remain too high. Anything over three minutes is usually too long, except maybe for the beginner walkers. The problem is that the longer the break between intervals, the more of an injury risk these will become because your muscles begin to "cool down" in between intervals. As with the other workouts in TEAMS, the goal is not to push yourself to the absolute limit, because the risk of injury at that point is too great. Also, we cannot emphasize enough that the first interval should always be the slowest of the day. As you progress through the repeats each repetition should get faster, just as when you are racing.

I remember one training session with Ecuador's Jefferson Perez, Olympic and three-time World Champion. Jefferson's workout consisted of eight one-mile intervals, each one faster than the previous. After warming up, he started off at 7:00 for his first mile. After a two-minute break he started again, completing the second mile in 6:30. By the seventh one he was walking 5:45, and his last mile was an amazing 5:37. This was typical of his workouts; his intervals always got faster from beginning to end. This was exactly how Jefferson raced, too.

25

Consider the 2003 IAAF World Championships in Paris, where Jefferson broke the 20km world record and earned a prize of $160,000. His first 10km was 39:10—very fast, but still 32 seconds behind Francisco "Paquillo" Fernandez of Spain, who pushed each kilometer faster and faster right from the start. Soon after 10km, Jefferson turned his trademark hat backward and made his move. He broke away from the chase pack and started to hunt down Paquillo with each passing step. By the time they hit 16km, Jefferson was gaining almost 10 seconds per kilometer on Paquillo. He came through the finish line in an amazing 1:17:21, winning his first World Championship in record time. How did he do this? By walking the second half of his race faster than the first, with a split of 38:11 for his second 10km. By accelerating in training, he taught his body how to accelerate when he raced.

Sample Speed Workouts

Here are some examples of speedwork sessions. Please remember that the total number of repeats should depend on your level of experience and stage of training.

Speed Distance: 200m	Heart Rate Based Pace: Zone #3 or #4	Level: Beginner
Rest Time: 2 minutes	Speed Based Pace: Zone #3 or #4	# of Intervals: 8 - 15
	Lactate Based Pace: > = 4.5 mmol/L	
Notes: This is great for beginner walkers or for youth walkers.		
Speed Distance: 400m	Heart Rate Based Pace: Zone #3 or #4	Level: Beginner to Moderate
Rest Time: 2 minutes	Speed Based Pace: Zone #3 or #4	# of Intervals: 8 to 15
	Lactate Based Pace: > = 4.5 mmol/L	
Notes: A great workout for beginner walkers or for those trying to fine tune their speed before a short distance race.		
Speed Distance: 800m	Heart Rate Based Pace: Zone #3 to #4	Level: Beginner to Moderate
Rest Time: 2 minutes	Speed Based Pace: Zone #3	# of Intervals: 8 to 12
	Lactate Based Pace: 3.0 to 4.5 mmol/L	
Notes: A great workout for beginner walkers to junior walkers trying to build up their speed.		
Speed Distance: 1km	Heart Rate Based Pace: Zone #3	Level: Moderate to Advanced
	Speed Based Pace: Zone #3	
Rest Time: 2 minutes	Lactate Based Pace: 3.0 to 4.5 mmol/L	# of Intervals: 6 to 20
Notes: A solid workout for youth walkers to elite athletes.		
Speed Distance: 2km	Heart Rate Based Pace: Zone #3	Level: Moderate to Advanced
	Speed Based Pace: Zone #3	
Rest Time: 2 minutes	Lactate Based Pace: 3.0 to 4.5 mmol/L	# of Intervals: 4 to 8
Notes: This is a favorite of Olympic Champion Jefferson Perez. He did these repeatedly the year he broke the World Record.		
Speed Distance: 3km	Heart Rate Based Pace: Zone #3	Level: Moderate to Advanced
	Speed Based Pace: Zone #3	
Rest Time: 2 min	Lactate Based Pace: 3.0 to 4.5 mmol/L	# of Intervals: 3 to 6
Notes: This is a favorite of Andreas "Dre" Gustafsson of Sweden.		

Speed Distance: 4km	Heart Rate Based Pace: Zone #2 or #3	Level: Advanced
Rest Time: 2 min	Speed Based Pace: Zone #2 or #3	# of Intervals: 2 to 4
	Lactate Based Pace: 2.0 to 4.0 mmol/L	

Notes: This is a favorite workout of mine when I am in the In Season Racing phase.

Speed Distance: 5km	Heart Rate Based Pace: Zone #2 or #3	Level: Advanced
Rest Time: 2 min	Speed Based Pace: Zone #2 or #3	# of Intervals: 2 to 4
	Lactate Based Pace: 2.0 to 4.0 mmol/L	

Notes: This is for the advanced walker during the Late Season Base phase or during the In Season phase.

Speed Distance: 8km	Heart Rate Based Pace: Zone #2	Level: Advanced
Rest Time: 2 min	Speed Based Pace: Zone #2	# of Intervals: 2 to 4
	Lactate Based Pace: 2.0 to 3.0 mmol/L	

Notes: This is a great workout for those athletes training for the 20km or 50km, but they should not be taken lightly.

Speed Distance: 10km	Heart Rate Based Pace: Zone #2	Level: Advanced
Rest Time: 3 min	Speed Based Pace: Zone #2	# of Intervals: 2
	Lactate Based Pace: 2.0 to 3.0 mmol/L	

Notes: A great workout for the marathon or if you are training for the 50km.

Speed Distance: 5km, 4km, 3km, 2km ,1km	Heart Rate Based Pace: Zone #3	Level: Advanced
	Speed Based Pace: Zone #3	
Rest Time: 2 minutes	Lactate Based Pace: 3.0 to 4.5 mmol/L	# of Intervals: 1

Notes: A great 20km workout!

Mexican Speedwork

Speed Distance: 1000m, 800m, 600m, 400m, 200m	Heart Rate Based Pace: Zone #3 or #4	Level: Beginner to Advanced
	Speed Based Pace: Zone #3 or #4	
	Lactate Based Pace: 3.0 to >=4.5 mmol/L	
Rest Time: 2 min to 1:15		# of Intervals: 2 to 4

Notes: This workout was named when Curt Clausen, Philip Dunn and I were in Poland training with the Mexican team who were there under the direction of Professor Hauslabor. Start off walking 1000m in Zone #3 or Zone #4, then take 2 minutes rest, then walk an 800m with a 1:45 rest, then walk a 600m taking 1:30 rest, then walk a 400m taking 1:15 rest, then walk 200m and take a 2 minute rest before starting over again with the next set. Once you do this workout, you are going to love it as a way to fine tune your speed before your shorter distance competitions.

Andrew Special

Speed Distance: 1km, 2km, 3km, 3km, 2km, 1km	Heart Rate Based Pace: Zone #3	Level: Moderate to Advanced
	Speed Based Pace: Zone #3	
Rest Time: 2 minutes	Lactate Based Pace: 3.0 to 4.5 mmol/L	# of Intervals: 1

Notes: This workout was a favorite of 2000 Olympian Andrew Hermann as a great way to sharpen up his legs after long periods of 50km training. It is also known as a ladder.

Tempo Workouts

Tempo workouts are a great way to get in shape quickly. However, sometimes if done too frequently or at too fast of a pace, they can cause more harm than good. Therefore, you must be careful with this type of training. The TEAMS philosophy calls for very few of these workouts.

Tempo workouts are training sessions in which the athlete warms up, walks a distance of 5km to 15km in Zone #2 or Zone #3 and then does the cool down. They are valuable to gauge fitness if an athlete has not raced for a long time, or to see how well the athlete is adapting to training. Generally, however, I prefer to do my Zone #3 training in spurts, as with fartleks, because they get the body accustomed to race pace without taxing the body as much. Since fartleks are broken into parts, they permit you to walk a longer distance at a faster pace than tempo workouts.

Another danger of tempo workouts is athletes walking this workout together in a group are often tempted to turn it into a mini-race, trying to outdo their partners and win the workout. **Racing is for competitions, not for training.** Many athletes in such a training setting would come to dread their weekly tempo "races" and would break down mentally as the season progressed; when the big peak races of the season came around, they had nothing left in their mental or physical banks. Jeff Salvage recalls when he was training seriously, his Coach Gary Westerfield would require athletes to do extra miles if they went too fast. This is one way to combat the racing mentality.

Some training philosophies suggest one tempo workout per week. *Race Walk like a Champion* includes tempo workouts during certain phases of training, but limits both the speed and distance of these workouts to manageable levels. This can work, especially if you train alone, where the temptation to race the workout is less intense, and if you have no midseason races to test yourself. Although this might work for some athletes, I feel the amount of training mileage necessary to be a high-quality athlete in long-distance racing, limits the number of straight tempo workouts required.

Some coaches refer to tempo workouts as "time trials," but this is really a mislabeling. Time trials are simulated races and are thus at a much higher intensity than tempo workouts. The TEAMS system does not include time trials—unless you count actual races as time trials. We exclude them because they typically require a decrease in mileage before and after the trial. For example, if an athlete does a 3km time trial in preparation for an upcoming 5km race, we believe a fartlek workout such as 3 x 1km/500 or 5 x 1km/500m would be preferable since the athlete will get a longer workout in this way and reduce recovery time besides. Generally, we believe that fartleks provide better speed endurance training than tempo workouts and are much more prudent than time trials.

Progression Walks

Though also rarely used in the TEAMS system of training, progression walks have value for a beginner athlete or when one is transitioning from the earlier to the later phase of base work, as we explain further in chapter 3.

In a progression walk an athlete race walks a certain portion, perhaps half, of the total workout distance in Zone #1, then gradually starts to increase the pace by a few seconds per kilometer, or per mile, until the last portion of the walk is completed at about Zone #2 pace.

Progression walks are good for getting athletes moving again after long periods of base work doing easy walks, or to help an athlete regain confidence in his or her abilities after some time off or an injury.

Technique Drills - Stretching - Cross Training

One does not develop great technique solely by race walking. Technique drills before working out, as well as stretching and strength training after workouts, will help your body improve its range of motion, flexibility and strength so that you can maintain ideal race walking technique.

Technique drills are an ideal way for you to warm up before your walking workout. They will not specifically be shown in the training schedules, but you should always perform them. This is especially important for beginner and masters athletes. While we would like you to reach this lofty goal, if your time is limited, make sure you perform them at least three times per week Similarly, stretching should be performed after every workout as a cool-down. Strength training, in contrast, should be performed no more than two or three days a week.

In *Race Walk Clinic - in a Book* we prescribed drills, stretches, and exercises based upon specific problems in your technique. Here we will simply identify drills, stretches, and strength training exercises that are useful for all race walkers attempting to develop good race walking technique. For a complete description of each exercise, please see *Race Walk Clinic - in a Book* or www.racewalk.com.

Technique Drills

A paradigm shift in training methodology has occurred over the last 20 years. Back in the 1980s static stretches were generally recommended to improve flexibility. Now dynamic flexibility drills, technique drills, are recognized as the key to increased range of motion, flexibility, and efficient race walking technique. Technique drills should be performed before working out and as a regular part of your warm-up routine. You do not need to perform every technique drill, just the ones that focus on your specific requirements.

 LONG STRIDES - LONG ARMS DRILL

Purpose: To improve forward hip rotation as well as to help beginning walkers develop a feel for what proper hip rotation feel like.

Duration: 30 meters.

 HURDLERS DRILL

Purpose: To improve hip range of motion.

Duration: 10 - 15 repetitions per leg.

FORWARD LEG KICK DRILL

Purpose: To improve hip range of motion.

Duration: 10 - 15 repetitions per leg.

 ## SIDE LEG SWING DRILL

Purpose: To improve hip range of motion.

Duration: 10 - 15 repetitions per leg.

 ## FOOT PLANT DRILL

Purpose: To help beginning walkers understand what a straightened knee feels like. More advanced walkers may skip this drill.

Duration: 10 - 15 repetitions per leg.

 ## BACKWARDS WINDMILL DRILL

Purpose: To improve range of motion in the shoulders, allowing them to be more relaxed.

Duration: 30 meters.

 ## BEND DOWN HAMSTRING DRILL

Purpose: To improve hamstring flexibility.

Duration: 30 meters.

 ## QUICK STEPS - HANDS BEHIND BACK DRILL

Purpose: To improve turnover and warm up the body.

Duration: 30 meters.

Stretching

Although stretching is no longer considered an ideal warm-up, it is an excellent cool-down activity and should be included as part of your post-workout regimen. In addition, if a particular area is sore, you may wish to stretch it after warming up completely. Stretching a cold muscle is not recommended as it can do more damage than good.

TRADITIONAL HAMSTRING STRETCH

Purpose: To improve hamstring flexibility.

Duration: 20 - 30 seconds per stretch. Repeat 2-3 times per leg.

IMPROVED TOE TOUCHING HAMSTRING STRETCH

Purpose: To improve hamstring flexibility.

Duration: 20 - 30 seconds, switch foot position and repeat.

TRADITIONAL CALF STRETCH

Purpose: To improve outer calf flexibility.

Duration: 20 - 30 seconds for each leg.

BENT KNEE CALF STRETCH

Purpose: To improve inner calf flexibility.

Duration: 20 - 30 seconds for each leg. This exercise can be started as the Traditional Calf Stretch is completed.

ADVANCED CALF STRETCH

Purpose: To improve outer calf flexibility.

Duration: 20 - 30 seconds for each leg.

SEATED SHIN STRETCH

Purpose: To improve shin flexibility; this exercise also helps with shin splints.

Duration: 20 - 30 seconds for each shin.

TIM'S STRETCH

Purpose: To improve hip flexor flexibility.

Duration: 20 - 30 seconds for each leg.

IT BAND STRETCH

Purpose: To improve IT band flexibility.

Duration: 10 times for each side.

PIRIFORMIS STRETCH

Purpose: To improve flexibility in the piriformis, which can tighten from a race walker's hip rotation.

Duration: 20 to 30 seconds, 2 to 3 repetitions per leg .

 ## PRAYER STRETCH

Purpose: To stretch the lower back.

Duration: 30 seconds.

 ## ADVANCED SIDE STRETCH

Purpose: To improve forward hip rotation.

Duration: 2-3 times on each side.

Strength Training

Ideally one gets stronger from race walking. This is especially true if you can walk on a moderately rolling course of gentle hills. If not, or if you have strength deficiencies, then the following set of exercises can be a valuable addition to your training plan. Be aware that strength training late in the season or in the week just before a race is ill-advised. Similarly, there is no place for heavy weights or small numbers of repetitions in race walk training.

 ## STRAIGHT LEG RAISE EXERCISE

Purpose: To strengthen the muscles of the knee.

Duration: 15 times with each leg.

 ## WALK ON YOUR HEELS EXERCISE

Purpose: To strengthen the shins.

Duration: 30 meters.

 ## TOE RAISE EXERCISE

Purpose: To strengthen the shins.

Duration: Until your shins begin to fatigue; do not overdo.

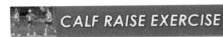 **CALF RAISE EXERCISE**

Purpose: To strengthen the calf muscles.

Duration: 10 - 15 times with each leg.

 LEG EXTENSION WITH MACHINE EXERCISE

Purpose: To strengthen the quadriceps muscles.

Duration: 2 - 3 sets of 10 - 15 repetitions per leg.

 LEG CURL WITH MACHINE EXERCISE

Purpose: To strengthen the hamstring muscles.

Duration: 2 - 3 sets of 10 - 15 repetitions per leg.

 CLAM SHELL EXERCISE

Purpose: To strengthen the hip abductors and thereby prevent your hip from dropping excessively.

Duration: 2 - 3 sets of 10 repetitions with each leg.

 BRIDGE WITH BALL EXERCISE

Purpose: To strengthen the lower back and upper hamstrings.

Duration: 2 sets of 15 times each.

 ALTERNATE ARM AND LEG EXERCISE

Purpose: To strengthen the lower back, glutes, upper hamstrings, and shoulders.

Duration: 2 sets of 10 repetitions.

TRADITIONAL STOMACH CRUNCHES

Purpose: To strengthen the core.

Duration: Hold for 3 seconds, up to 100 crunches.

BICYCLE EXERCISE

Purpose: To strengthen the core.

Duration: 25 cycles.

Purpose: For race walking specific overall arm strengthening.

Duration: 2 to 10 minutes.

Alternative Training Ideas

In addition, here are a few alternative training ideas for those that desire to cross train. Cross training is a great way to get in shape after coming back from an injury and it is a great way to get more aerobic work in without putting too much stress on your legs. For elite walkers, we sometimes prescribe second workouts in the same day as a walking workout. This is often in the form of an alternative exercise similar to those that follow:

Aqua Jogging

Sometimes as a form of cross-training we recommend "aqua jogging," which involves putting a floatable belt around your waist and running in the water. This is indicated by an "AJ" on the forthcoming training schedules. It is a great way to build strength and endurance during the base work phase and it is a great recovery tool also.

Elliptical

Utilizing an Elliptical machine is a great second workout to keep the stress off of your legs while still getting the cardiovascular work needed to keep improving. Kjersti Plaetzer utilized this to perfection as she came back from the birth of her second child and couldn't put too must stress on her knees.

Combining Walking with Running

One of the distinctive aspects of the TEAMS race walk training system is the inclusion of recovery runs. TEAMS uses these runs as a way to recover from race walk workouts, which may overtax some previously underutilized muscle groups. It is also easier on the mind than focusing on race walking technique in every workout. In addition, running some recovery workouts allows for a nice run in the forest, on a dirt trail, or along the beach to break up the boredom. Be careful to keep these runs as recovery work, do not push the pace.

While helpful for most walkers, easy runs are not appropriate for everyone. Walkers who have experienced running injuries should avoid the scheduled runs and replace them with easy Zone #1 walks, aqua jogging, or use of an elliptical machine.

Chapter Three: Developing a Schedule

Basic Philosophy

The TEAMS coaching philosophy is based on a simple fiscal analogy that Coach Stephan Plaetzer of Norway first explained to me. He said:

> "You can withdraw from the bank only what you have deposited into the bank or gained in interest, but you must time your withdrawals very carefully."

What Plaetzer meant is that endurance training is like a bank account. You must first make a deposit in your training account before you can withdraw from it. If your deposits are held longer, interest is gained. Then, when you ultimately withdraw your resources, you will have more than your initial deposit. If you frequently or immediately withdraw what you deposit, you'll never build a balance and have nothing to withdraw when you most need it – at race time.

It is imperative you make as many deposits into the bank as possible, so when the big race arrives your body can withdraw enough *energy* to perform at its best. Here are some good ways to make deposits into your bank:

- Properly paced endurance zone workouts.
- Properly paced speed endurance workouts.
- Proper recovery from speed endurance workouts.
- Proper nutrition.
- Proper sleep.
- Technique drills.
- Cooling down properly.

Conversely, mistakes like walking your workouts too fast, improper nutrition and sleep, and inadequate recovery time can withdraw "money" from your bank when you should be building up your account balance for the big race. Your balance will determine whether your body peaks when it counts, or if it will crash and burn after the first race of the season.

Proper Recovery

When you do your endurance workouts too fast, you hinder your body's ability to recover from the harder training days. Excessively fast endurance workouts cause athletes to peak too early in the season and can often lead to injury. Many times just as poorly trained walkers feel they are in the best shape of their life, they get injured. More likely than not, it was due to bouncing a check from the body bank. If you withdraw more than you have in your account by overtraining, you will become fatigued, injured, or both. Be smart and patient. Aim for consistency of training, not an instant solution. That is the key.

Properly paced speed-endurance workouts also add to your account balance because they allow your body to adapt to the harder training days. If you push your body to the brink of destruction by walking too fast, your body eventually pushes back and you will be unable to attain your training and performance goals.

As I prepared for my first Olympic Games, I started down a path full of repercussions for months to follow. I had nine weeks between the 20km Olympic Trials in Sacramento and the Olympic Games in Sydney, Australia. My coach set up a plan for me to do my best at the biggest race of my life. Virtually every other day we did speedwork repetitions for three weeks before the race. We had nine hard workouts during those three weeks, including a 1:25:55 20 km just 9 days before my race. Every other day I withdrew money from my bank. I did repetition after repetition. You can guess what happened. As I was doing my last hard workout, 10 x 1km, in the Olympic Village, I got injured. All that hard work went down the tubes in an instant. I had one of my most disappointing days in my athletic life, because I did not allow my body to recover from my harder training sessions.

Proper Nutrition

Proper nutrition is a complicated topic on which whole books have been written. We do not claim to be nutrition experts and therefore will not prescribe in detail the nutritional requirements for race walkers. It should be obvious that untested fads, fast food binges, and low calorie diets have no place in a race walker's nutritional repertoire. High carbohydrate diets with sufficient protein to rebuild muscles are the key to success.

You may be tempted to take nutritional supplements to round out your diet, but be aware that you can't always guarantee what you are ingesting in pill form. The Food and Drug Administration (FDA) does not monitor supplements in any way. When you rely on what the manufacturer states on the label, you are taking a risk—and if you are an elite athlete subject to drug testing you are taking a huge and unnecessary risk. The exact ingredients are not always listed on supplement labels. We prefer to see athletes get their vitamins from the foods they eat.

If you don't eat properly and you continue to train hard, your body will break down and you will get injured or sick. Every week of quality training that you miss is two percent of the year—and that two percent could make the difference between winning the race and failing to finish. You don't want your bank taking two percent of your savings account away each week, do you?

If you would like additional information on nutrition, a great resource is *Racing Weight* by Matt Fitzgerald. He has done a great job explaining how to get lean for peak performance.

Racing

Although hard races without proper recovery decrease our account balance, that does not mean you should avoid racing. In fact, racing is an important part of our training philosophy, because your ultimate goal is of course to race fast. However, you should avoid scheduling too many hard races over a short period of time, and you should give your body ample time to recover from each race. Too many coaches have their athletes walk a hard workout on the Tuesday after a Sunday race, just because they always have hard workouts on Tuesdays. This is very dangerous, especially after longer races. Don't add to your risk of injury in an attempt to gain an extra day of training. Be smart, rest properly, you've earned it.

Consistency of Training

Chapter 2 introduced the different types of workouts in the TEAMS philosophy. We will now put them together to develop a training schedule. It is not enough just to know the different types of workouts; instead you must schedule them in a logical way so that you peak properly. Our main theme will be **Consistency of Training**. This was one of the most important lessons I learned from my time with Team Plaetzer. If you are having great workouts one day and terrible workouts the next, you are teaching your body and mind to be inconsistent. In contrast, continual, consistent buildup of strong training is best suited to produce a gold medal performance.

When developing a schedule using the TEAMS system, you should determine what your most important race of the season is and work backwards from there. In this way you can figure out how many weeks to devote to each phase and how much racing you can do in preparation for peaking. Your biggest race may be a national or international championship; along the way you should place other races in the schedule so that you are tested and challenged but not exhausted.

Chapters 4 through 10 contain sample schedules tailored to specific groups of athletes. We have placed sample races directly into the schedule during weeks that they would typically fall. For example, youth athletes may aim to excel at the Penn Relays, the National Scholastic Indoor Championships, or the USATF Junior Nationals. Collegians attending NAIA schools may use their indoor and outdoor championships to prepare themselves for the USATF Indoor Championships (5,000m for men and 3,000m for women) and Outdoor Championships (20km). Elite athletes looking to walk wearing red, white and blue as they enter the Olympic Stadium, may seek to peak at the Olympic Trials, or at a race in Europe to meet the Olympic qualifying time standards. If they are strong enough to have locked in a spot early enough on the Olympic Team, they could even peak directly for the Olympic Games. Masters athletes have many choices, including the World Outdoor Masters Championships, World Indoor Masters Championships, or the Summer National Senior Games. In addition, masters athletes often chase after various national titles and age group records. When Jack Starr, Jeff Salvage's masters prodigy, was asked what distance he was targeting, Jack simply stated, "all of them." It is important to choose. The key is to target the most important races and set your goals around them. Fill in with other races, but be careful not to add too many. You can't peak for every race.

Injuries

One of the most foolish ways for an athlete to fail to accomplish his or her goals is by stubbornly attempting to complete every workout as it was planned weeks or months before. Schedules must be adapted for injuries, weather, or any other outside factors that could impact the athlete's training. For example, if you are just beginning to feel symptoms of an injury, you must alter the schedule to avoid worsening the problem. Sometimes you may push through just to be the tough guy, or for fear of getting out of shape. This could cause a major stress fracture or tear your hamstring. Don't let those few extra kilometers walked end up sapping your account balance. Injuries lead to inconsistent training, which in turn can cause more injuries and worse athletic performances.

Upon returning from an injury, always wait an extra day or two before trying to get back to your regular training, to make sure that your injury has fully healed. Too many times athletes rush to get in shape for their next race, only to be back on the sidelines with another injury caused by compensating for the original injury. Take a few extra days of cross training before returning to race walking again. That is one of the keys to being consistent with your training.

Periodic Training

In the TEAMS system of training we vary the workouts for each day of the week in patterns based upon how far along you are in your training schedule. The TEAMS system of training is periodic and usually has four main phases:

- Phase I - Early Season Base Work
- Phase II - Late Season Base Work
- Phase III – In Season Racing
- Phase IV - Peak Season

Phase I - Early Season Base Work

As with any structure, a strong base is essential if you wish to build up for end-of-the-season success. The exact formation of the base should vary based upon the athlete's performance level and ability to stay focused. Don't ask young kids to endure a 12 to 16 week Base phase like an Olympic-level athlete; they will get bored and find something else to do very quickly.

In the Early Season Base Work phase, the goal is to gradually build up your mileage so that you reduce your risk of injury and to get your body ready for what is to come over the next few months. This is the period where you should really try to deposit as much as you can into the bank by concentrating on the Endurance Zone #1 workouts. These workouts are the key to staying strong throughout the season and to peaking when it counts. If you push these workouts too fast, you will peak far too early in the year and you will struggle in the big races later.

As you put more stress on your body with longer and harder workouts during the In Season Racing phase, any muscle imbalances will be exacerbated and will thus cause an injury risk. Trying to fix muscle weakness issues in the middle of the season is difficult. Therefore, one must fix them now. Incorporating traditional weight exercises of high reps and low weight can help. However, this can result in a shortening of the muscles at a time when you are trying to achieve a maximum range of motion. Therefore, during the Early Season Base Work phase you must always be working on both your flexibility and range of motion drills, as illustrated in *Race Walk Clinic* - *in a Book* and prescribed in chapter 2. Attaining greater flexibility can improve your technique by allowing you to walk through a full range of motion. The better your range of motion, the more efficient you become and the more you get out of every step.

38

The Early Season Base Work phase for most groups of walkers should last about 6 to 8 weeks, more for elite athletes, and of course less for the youth. Here is the structure for a schedule for a typical training week during this phase:

Monday	Tuesday	Wednesday	Thursday	Friday	Saturday	Sunday
Shorter Distance Zone #1 Walk	Shorter Distance Zone #1 Walk or Cross Training	Longer Distance Zone #1 Walk	OFF or short distance Zone #1 Walk	Shorter Distance Zone #1 Walk	Longer Distance Zone #1 Walk	Hiking

This generic example is intentionally vague; chapters 4 through 10 fill in the suggested workout lengths and other details for every level of athlete.

Focus on Technique

In addition to completing the prescribed distance, race walkers must focus on high-quality technique during every workout. Time must be taken to do technique drills and mobility exercises so that you can increase the range of motion of your hips, hamstrings, calves, shoulders, and lower back.

Every day is a technique day for race walkers utilizing the TEAMS system, especially during the Early Season Base Work phase. Walkers must review regularly a mental checklist of what good technique looks like. They should start from the top of the body and work their way down, asking themselves these questions:

- Is my head straight and in a neutral position? Having your head, which typically weighs about eight pounds, leaning to one side, or leaning down, is going to cause an injury or muscle imbalance to occur. Care must be taken to keep it straight.
- How are my shoulders? Are they up by my ears or nice and low? Your shoulders should be as low as possible. When you keep them low, your center of gravity lowers and your arms are freed to swing with less resistance.
- How are my arms? Your arms should be able to swing like a pendulum on a clock. You should keep a relatively constant angle at about 90 degrees between your upper and lower arm at the elbow, and they should not be pumping. Care should be taken so that the hands trace a few inches behind your hips and to the height of your sternum, the center of your chest, in the front.
- How are my knees? Ask yourself if your knees are straightened upon heel contact with the ground. Are they driving upward instead of staying low to the ground? Knees that drive high lead to the risk of disqualification and inefficient walking.
- How are my feet? Your swing foot should be as low to the ground as possible as it swings forward. When the heel of the swing foot makes contact with the ground in front of the body, the foot angle to the ground should be between 20 and 25 degrees.

Of course, only focus on one aspect of race walking technique at a time.

Phase II - Late Season Base Work

After about six to eight weeks of the Early Season Base Work phase, you should be ready to move to the next phase. Having completed enough endurance base training workouts, sufficient range of motion drills, and stretching, your body and mind are ready for the next step. It is important to note that shifting to a new phase does not relieve you from performing flexibility and range of motion training. Instead, we start to use our increased mobility from the drills and stretches, as well as adding some fartleks to the training regimen, to gradually adapt the body to walking faster paces. The duration of the workouts lengthens as well. Ideally, we wish to build strength naturally and in a sport specific manner. The best way to do this is to incorporate hill work into your longer distance days. If you live in a hilly area, you can start to incorporate more challenging courses with gradual hills.

Since this phase typically occurs during the winter, it can also include a few short indoor races. You will be amazed at how fast you can walk even without doing the traditional weeks of speed repetitions prescribed by most training programs. I have had the privilege of winning the infamous Millrose Games race walk, a one-mile sprint in New York's Madison Square Garden, six times in my career. My fastest time of 5:46 was achieved in the year when I did the least amount of fast walking. Jeff Salvage had a similar result, walking his one-mile PR while he was training for the 50km. Our feats were accomplished with a large volume of quality base work and some longer intervals, which, when done properly, raise the ceiling of one's lactate threshold. This builds a nice strong engine to rev up when the gun goes off on the start line.

> "The Foundation Period (what we call the Early and Late Season Base phase) of your training year has the largest effect on the height of your peak. This is the period of the year that focuses on building the superior aerobic engine that will power the rest of your energy systems." -- Chris Carmichael, Coach of Lance Armstrong

The Late Season Base Work phase typically lasts about six to eight weeks for an elite level athlete. Here is the structure for a schedule of a typical training week during the Late Season Base Work phase:

Monday	Tuesday	Wednesday	Thursday	Friday	Saturday	Sunday
Shorter Distance Zone #1 Walk	Fartlek	Longer Distance Zone #1 Walk	OFF or shorter distance Zone #1 Walk	Shorter Distance Zone #1 Walk	Longer Distance Zone #1 Walk	Hiking

When we begin giving more detailed schedules you will see multiple components in some of the boxes. A warm-up period is denoted as "w-up" and the cool down period is denoted as "c-d." In the following example, the complete workout consists of a 3km warm-up, a 5km in Zone #2, followed by a 1 km in Zone #1 with the 5km/1km segment repeated twice. Finally you walk a 2km cool down.

3km w-u
Fartlek 2 x 5km /1km
Zone #2
2km c-d

Phase III – In Season Racing Phase

The third phase lasts from 12 to 20 weeks for an Olympic-level athlete. For other athletes it may vary depending on the duration of their season, but it should be the longest single phase of training in the season. The goal of this phase is to push your lactate threshold higher while still walking enough mileage to maintain your strength through the end of the season.

Since Phase III contains more stress in the form of faster workouts, it is important to focus on recovering from the harder days. Most coaches tell their athletes to focus primarily on the faster days, but we believe that how well the athlete *recovers* from those harder days will determine his or her consistency. This string of successful weeks of training will produce a champion.

The structural change in the schedule from Phase II to Phase III is the additional fartlek workout per week. Now, one fartlek day comprises longer intervals and the other day comprises shorter intervals. Shorter, of course, is relative. We do not mean to imply really short intervals such as 200 meters. One example of a fartlek in the TEAMS system of training is 5 x 2km/1km on the longer fartlek day. In this fartlek, an athlete walks 2km in Zone # 3 and 1km in Zone #1 and repeats this sequence a total of five times. Then, the shorter day might be 1km/500m or 500m/500m, or even the Spanish fartlek of 800m/400m. More than likely, a favorite of many of the athletes is the Norwegian Fartlek, especially the 2010 U.S. Indoor National Champion Maria Michta. It consists of eight fast segments of one to eight minutes at Zone #3, in the order of 2-4-6-8-7-5-3-1, with a two-minute Zone #1 walk in between.

One key to successful training is to continuously mix up the distances so that your body and mind are constantly taxed and forced to adapt. Many training books use a progression in which you do a few more intervals each week, but in which the intervals are always the same length. That system may be good for some athletes, but it causes others, including myself, to get bored doing the same thing week after week. Mixing it up will keep an athlete's head in the game, and ready to fight when it counts.

Let us underscore once again that following this training program properly requires more than pushing hard on the fartlek days. The most important aspect of training is to allow the body to absorb the hard days by walking the Zone #1 training sessions properly. If the recovery days are pushed too hard, then recovery will take longer than necessary, especially after a race. Since there will usually be various races during this phase, the athlete must recover as quickly as possible from each race. The best way to do this is to avoid rushing right back into harder workouts without a sufficient number of easier days.

Here is the structure for a schedule for one week of the In Season Racing phase.

Monday	Tuesday	Wednesday	Thursday	Friday	Saturday	Sunday
Shorter Distance Zone #1 Walk	Longer Fartlek Zone #2 / #3	Longer Distance Zone #1 Walk	Off or Medium Distance Zone #1 Walk	Shorter Distance Zone #1 Walk	Shorter Fartlek Zone #3 / #4	Longer Distance Zone #1 Walk

Phase IV – Peak Season

This is the time when all the hard work comes together. This phase typically lasts for just four to six weeks. It is when you put forth your best performance of the year and all of your hard work pays off. As always, recovery from the harder training days is crucial. You must also focus on eating well and getting plenty of sleep so your hard work does not go to waste.

The Peak phase features a gradual decrease in the number of fartleks and an increase in the amount of speedwork sessions, but still never more than two times per week. In addition, the overall mileage decreases to help the legs feel fresh and ready to fight. The structure for a schedule of a sample week in the Peak phase follows.

Monday	Tuesday	Wednesday	Thursday	Friday	Saturday	Sunday
Shorter Distance Zone #1 Walk	Longer speed repeats Zone #3	Medium Distance Zone #1 Walk	Off or Short Distance Zone #1 Walk	Shorter Distance Zone #1 Walk	Shorter speed repeats Zone #3 or Zone #4	Medium Distance Zone #1 Walk

Usually Phase IV has one goal: to succeed in the most important race of the year. The mind and body have prepared all season for this moment. Along with continuing good physical training, you must take into account how you respond to pressure. Some people need extra pressure to excel, while others crumble under its weight. You need to know how to balance seriousness and relaxation at this point. Dr. Jim Bauman, the U.S. Olympic Training Center's sports psychologist, used to tell us to "have a good race," while everyone else around us would say "have a great race." When I asked him why he never told us to have a "great" race, he said that we had enough internal pressure to perform well and didn't need any more pressure from the outside. His words were very wise.

Another point of psychology: while I was trying to qualify for the 2004 Olympic Games, Coach Stephan Plaetzer taught me that it would be just me and the road—nothing else mattered. He instilled in me not to be distracted by the crowd, the competition, or anything else because no one else could carry me through as the clock ticked slowly toward 1 hour and 23 minutes, the time I needed to beat in order to clinch a spot on the Olympic team. Fortunately, I listened well and achieved my goal walking a time of 1:22:02 to break the American Road Record.

By this point in the season, an athlete may have logged hundreds, if not thousands, of training miles and spent thousands of dollars on airfare, lodging, and car rentals for the season's races. Don't let that hard work and money go down the drain. Prepare yourself physically and mentally for your biggest challenge of the season.

Alternative Schedules

We recognize that not every athlete wants to, or is able to, train every day. So here are some examples of how to structure the TEAMS program with less frequent training. You should be able to use these to develop a schedule tailored to your personal life situation.

Three Days a Week of Training:

Early Season Base Work

Monday	Tuesday	Wednesday	Thursday	Friday	Saturday	Sunday
OFF	Medium Distance walk Zone #1	OFF	Medium distance walk Zone #1	OFF	Longer distance walk Zone #1	OFF

Late Season Base Work

Monday	Tuesday	Wednesday	Thursday	Friday	Saturday	Sunday
OFF	Longer fartlek Zone #2	OFF	Medium distance walk Zone #1	OFF	Longer distance walk Zone #1	OFF

In Season Racing

Monday	Tuesday	Wednesday	Thursday	Friday	Saturday	Sunday
OFF	Longer Fartlek Zone #2 / #3	OFF	OFF	Shorter Fartlek Zone #3/ #4	OFF	Longer distance walk Zone #1

Peak Season

Monday	Tuesday	Wednesday	Thursday	Friday	Saturday	Sunday
OFF	Short Repetitions Zone #3 / #4	OFF	OFF	Short Repetitions Zone #3 / #4	OFF	Medium distance walk Zone #1

Four Days a Week of Training:

Early Season Base Work

Monday	Tuesday	Wednesday	Thursday	Friday	Saturday	Sunday
OFF	Medium distance walk Zone #1	OFF	Medium distance walk Zone #1	OFF	Longer distance walk Zone #1	Long hike

Late Season Base Work

Monday	Tuesday	Wednesday	Thursday	Friday	Saturday	Sunday
OFF	Medium distance walk Zone #1	OFF	Medium distance walk Zone #1	OFF	Longer fartlek Zone #2	Longer distance walk Zone #1

In Season Racing

Monday	Tuesday	Wednesday	Thursday	Friday	Saturday	Sunday
OFF	Longer fartlek Zone #2 / #3	OFF	Medium distance walk Zone #1	OFF	Shorter fartlek Zone #3 / #4	Longer distance walk Zone #1

Peak Season

Monday	Tuesday	Wednesday	Thursday	Friday	Saturday	Sunday
OFF	Medium repetitions Zone #3	OFF	Medium distance walk Zone #1	OFF	Shorter Repetitions Zone #3 / #4	Medium distance walk Zone #1

Five Days a Week of Training:

Early Season Base Work

Monday	Tuesday	Wednesday	Thursday	Friday	Saturday	Sunday
OFF	Shorter distance walk Zone #1	Medium distance walk Zone #1	Shorter distance walk Zone #1	OFF	Longer distance walk Zone #1	Long hike

Late Season Base Work

Monday	Tuesday	Wednesday	Thursday	Friday	Saturday	Sunday
OFF	Shorter distance walk Zone #1	Medium/long distance walk Zone #1	Shorter distance walk Zone #1	OFF	Longer fartlek Zone #2	Longer distance walk Zone #1

In Season Racing

Monday	Tuesday	Wednesday	Thursday	Friday	Saturday	Sunday
OFF	Longer Fartlek Zone #2 / #3	Medium distance walk Zone #1	Shorter distance walk Zone #1	OFF	Shorter fartlek Zone #3 / #4	Long distance walk Zone #1

Peak Season

Monday	Tuesday	Wednesday	Thursday	Friday	Saturday	Sunday
OFF	Medium or short speedwork Zone #3 / #4	Medium distance walk Zone #1	Shorter distance walk Zone #1	OFF	Shorter Repetitions Zone #3 / #4	Medium distance walk Zone #1

Tapering and Recovering from Races

Sometimes races occur at inconvenient times during your training schedule. If you consider a mid-season race important, you must taper and recovery properly. This entails gradually reducing the training demands placed on your body as the race approaches. Long-term success depends on proper tapering for the race and on proper recovery afterwards. Therefore, we demonstrate how to modify an existing schedule when you decide to add a race midseason. Here are some sample tapers and recovery weeks for various race distances.

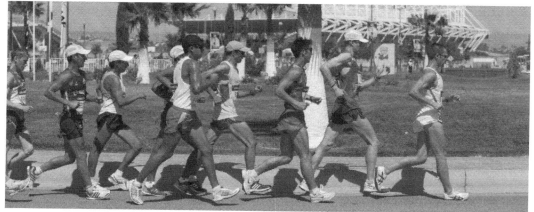

Lead Pack at the 2010 IAAF World Race Walking Cup

44

5km Race Taper and Recovery

Week	Monday	Tuesday	Wednesday	Thursday	Friday	Saturday	Sunday
1	Shorter distance walk Zone #1	Speedwork 2 or 3km warm-up 5 to 12 x 500m Zone #3 or Zone #4 90 sec rest 2km c-d (The # of repetitions depends on your level)	Medium distance walk Zone #1	Shorter distance walk Zone #1 or OFF	Shorter distance walk Zone #1	Very short distance walk Zone #1	5km race
2	Cross training or medium distance walk Zone #1	OFF	Medium distance walk Zone #1	Medium distance walk Zone #1	Shorter distance walk Zone #1	Medium distance Fartlek	Longer distance walk Zone #1

(Note the above program does not prescribe a hard workout until the sixth day after the race.)

10km Race Taper and Recovery

Week	Monday	Tuesday	Wednesday	Thursday	Friday	Saturday	Sunday
1	Medium distance walk Zone #1	Norwegian fartlek or 5 to 8 to 12 x 500m speedwork 90 seconds rest Zone #3	Medium distance walk Zone #1	Medium distance walk Zone #1 or OFF	Shorter distance walk Zone #1	Short distance walk Zone #1	10km race
2	Medium distance walk Zone #1	OFF	Medium distance walk Zone #1	Longer distance walk Zone #1	Shorter distance walk Zone #1	Medium distance fartlek	Longer distance walk Zone #1

20km Race Taper and Recovery

Week	Monday	Tuesday	Wednesday	Thursday	Friday	Saturday	Sunday
1	Medium distance walk Zone #1	Norwegian fartlek Zone #3	Medium distance walk Zone #1	OFF or short distance walk	Shorter distance walk Zone #1	Short distance walk Zone #1	20km race
2	Shorter distance walk Zone #1	Short distance walk Zone #1	OFF	Medium distance walk Zone #1	Shorter distance walk Zone #1	Shorter fartlek	Longer distance walk Zone #1

While many structures of schedules are proposed in this chapter, many more permutations still exist. Coaches constantly modify an athlete's schedule based up the individuality of the athlete, race schedules, and life issues that get in the way of following the ideal training program. Feel free to modify our prescription to success, but always keep in mind the guiding principles of your training account balance by depositing more than you withdraw.

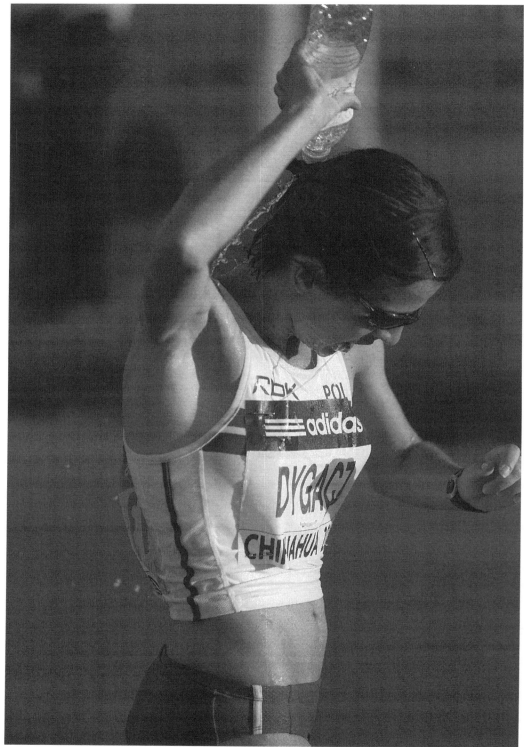

Agnieszka Dygacz trying to cool off during the 2010 IAAF Race Walking World Cup

Chapter Four: Race Walking for Youth

Like other athletic endeavors, race walking has enormous value for children. Belonging to a team increases a young athletes' self-esteem, helps them stay focused in school, and keeps them away from drugs and out of gangs. My involvement for the past seven years with the South Texas Walking Club, one of the nation's leaders in youth race walking, impressed upon me just how much race walking positively affects younger athletes.

America is plagued by an obesity epidemic, fueled by television, video games, and other electronic distractions. The prevalence of diabetes among children has skyrocketed in recent years. Race walking can help them stay in good shape and break hereditary chains of diabetes and other illnesses.

My favorite example is Alex Chavez from Pharr, Texas. Alex's family had a history of diabetes and he was smart enough to know, even at the age of 10, that he had to break the cycle. Athletics was the key, but he was afraid to try football, the most popular sport in Texas. As a result, he was delighted when introduced to race walking at his elementary school by Coach A.C. Jaime. Since that day Alex has lost almost 40 pounds and become a National Junior Olympic Champion, an AAU Junior Olympic record holder, and a High School Indoor National Champion. Alex broke the chains that threatened to bind him, and others can do the same.

Lessons for Working with the Youth

The goal of any coach of children is to provide a safe and positive environment. Coach A.C. Jaime is the embodiment of an ideal youth coach. A former mayor of Pharr, Coach Jaime is like a grandfather to many of his athletes, doing all that is in his power to help them develop. By working closely with A.C., I've learned many lessons about mentoring young athletes.

The first lesson, and the number one goal in youth sports, is to be able to smile and laugh before, during, and after each training session. Youngsters should not be just pounding out mile after mile. Coaches must make participating in race walking fun and allow them an opportunity to be kids. Childhood years are about being carefree while still learning the rules of life. Certainly, some of the workouts are hard, but enjoying the workout keeps it from becoming too difficult. The goal is to teach younger race walkers they can work hard and succeed while still enjoying themselves.

Another significant lesson is the importance of teaching proper technique. Learning to race walk legally, despite the temptation to run or to bend the knee prematurely, teaches self-discipline. If children learn bad habits by trying to walk faster than their technique allows at a young age, they form a faulty technical base that becomes hard to break later in life. Disciplining oneself to observe the rules of race walking pays huge dividends later, both on the track and in the classroom. Thus we teach good technique first and focus on becoming faster afterward. I believe that one reason the South Texas Walking Club has had a huge success is the time it spends on technique drills.

Stretching is also extremely important in preventing injuries and should be part of every cool down. Coach Jaime had already taught his club members proper stretching, but I made sure to reinforce this point. It never hurts to hear the same things from two different people! You can find many stretches and technique drills appropriate for youths in *Race Walk Clinic – in a Book*; we have provided a short list of some of the most important ones in chapter 2.

We do not provide a full 10-month training schedule for youths in this book, because they cannot stay focused for that long and should not be pushed to make race walking their sole focus. Rather, they should be encouraged to participate in as many sports as possible so they can develop the coordination required of a great all-around athlete. Single-focus athletic programs leave kids tired, burned out, and looking for something else to do. Don't treat them as if they are pros; keep the training fun and interactive so that they are more likely to enjoy practice and continue training into their teenage years. No 10-year-old has ever made an Olympic Track and Field team; we need to make race walking exciting for our 10-year-olds while they get stronger and faster to the point where perhaps someday they can become Olympians.

Here are some ideas for games to keep younger kids laughing as they train. Caution: always have the kids warm up properly first.

Duck Duck Goose. Younger kids love this classic game, so we make it a way for kids to have fun and walk fast at the same time. The rules of the game are the same as in the traditional version, except that when the person is making their way around the circle saying "duck, duck, duck, GOOSE!" they, along with the person who gets "goosed" must race walk around the circle. To make it fairer for the person getting up, and also to force the kids to race walk a little longer, we have the kids do two laps around the circle.

Freeze Tag – Again, follow the normal rules of this game, except that everyone must race walk rather than run. It helps to keep the playing field relatively small, because otherwise it is too difficult and not much fun for the tagger. You may also want to have more than one person be "it."

The Blob – This is a variation of freeze tag. One person starts as "it" and then attempts to tag someone else. Once tagged, both kids have to hold hands with each other while race walking around in pursuit of other people to tag. Once the group of "it's" (called a blob) reaches four, then the group can break up into pairs of two and try and catch the other kids. The bigger the group playing, the better this game works.

Kickball – Set up a small field and have everyone play traditional kickball, but instead of running the participants must race walk to each base or to field the ball. This might sound easy, but it is very difficult to tag someone out while race walking!

Relay Races - Most kids like to compete and competing with a team is even more fun. Therefore, do relay races of 100m or 200m instead of traditional interval training. The kids will enjoy it more, smile more, and get more out of it because they won't notice that they are training at the same time as they are having fun.

Developing a Training Schedule for Youth Race Walkers

Since the Junior Olympic program is our largest development program, our training schedule sets the national championship meets as the peak of the season and works backward from there. It is rare for youth walkers to focus on race walking for ten solid months, so this schedule is significantly shorter than the others provided in subsequent chapters. A coach can always choose to extrapolate this schedule to a longer, or shorter, duration if necessary.

Our youth training schedule starts about March 15, or about 20 weeks before the Junior Olympic Championships. Since most youths walk only during this season, they must start with very modest training during the first few weeks. Our schedule assumes that the youths were active in some manner, usually in other sports.

Early in the season, it is especially important to focus on technique to avoid potential disqualifications. When an athlete gets disqualified due to bad technique, not only do they get discouraged, but so do their parents who may have spent hundreds of dollars traveling to the association or regional championships. A coach who wants to keep athletes and parents motivated must take the time to focus on good technique.

I will never forget the year when I helped coach the South Texas Walking Club athletes in the two Junior Olympic Championships (USATF and AAU) on opposite coasts and told them how lucky they were to be able to go swimming in both the Pacific and the Atlantic oceans in the same summer. They were able to do that, not because some coach made them partake in long training sessions, but because they had a supportive network of people who cared about them.

When you are looking at the schedule, please be aware that the normal amount of time the kids do each phase is much shorter than more advanced athletes. Kids typically compete in short races of 1500m to 1-mile. At this age, a lot of "high quality mileage" only causes a loss of focus and interest. It has to be fun and exciting.

Phase I - Early Season Base Work for Youth Race Walkers

The Early Season Base Work phase for your athletes lasts just three weeks. If it lasts longer, there is a higher risk that the kids will get bored quickly and may not make it through the entire summer. The goal of this phase is to work on good technique and get the kids' bodies accustomed to race walking. Some of the athletes have never race walked before, and the others haven't done it since the previous August. Athletes must not do too much too soon, due to the risk of injury. The kids have probably grown a few inches since they last race walked and their physique has changed, so it is best to start off nice and easy and not put too much stress on their bodies. You will also notice there are two or three days off each week. Don't let the kids race walk every day; they have had too much time off to jump immediately into daily training. Also, make sure they perform the technique drills and stretching regularly.

Week	Monday	Tuesday	Wednesday	Thursday	Friday	Saturday	Sunday	Mileage
1	2km walk Zone #1	3km walk Zone #1	OFF	3km walk Zone #1	OFF	4km walk Zone #1	OFF	12km Total
2	3km walk Zone #1	3km walk Zone #1	OFF	3km walk Zone #1	OFF	5km walk Zone #1	OFF	14km Total
3	3km walk Zone #1	4km walk Zone #1	OFF	4km walk Zone #1	OFF	5km walk Zone #1	3km walk Zone #1	20km Total

Phase II - Late Season Base Work for Youth Race Walkers

The Late Season Base Work phase also lasts just three weeks. Here we include one relatively easy speed repeat or fartlek session per week to get the kids walking fast again. Make sure that the kids are performing their technique drills correctly and stretching properly. Remind them that the first interval of a speed workout should be the slowest and that each subsequent one should get a little faster. Remember, the athletes are trying to build a solid foundation for the rest of the season, so don't let the them push themselves to exhaustion at every workout.

Week	Monday	Tuesday	Wednesday	Thursday	Friday	Saturday	Sunday	Mileage
4	3km walk Zone #1	2km w-up Fartlek 6 x 100m/100m 1.5km c-d Zone #3	OFF	3km walk Zone #1	OFF	5km walk Zone #1	3km walk Zone #1	17.5km Total
5	3km walk Zone #1	2km w-up Fartlek 6 x 200/200 1.5km c-d Zone #3	OFF	3km walk Zone #1	OFF	6km walk Zone #1	4km walk Zone #1	20km Total
6	3km walk Zone #1	5km walk Zone #1	OFF	3km walk Zone #1	OFF	1.5km w-up Fartlek 4 x 400/400 1.5km c-d Zone #3	5km walk Zone #1	22km Total

Phase III - In Season Racing for Youth Race Walkers

Lasting nine weeks, the In Season Racing phase includes two harder sessions each week along with two days of longer training. During this phase young athletes should work on their speed and still have fun while getting ready for the big races later in the summer. As noted previously, do not overlook regularly performing technique drills and stretching. Again, note during speedwork or fartlek sessions the first interval should **always** be the slowest.

Week	Monday	Tuesday	Wednesday	Thursday	Friday	Saturday	Sunday	Mileage
7	3km walk Zone #1	Speedwork 2km w-up 4 x 800m 3:00 rest 1.5km c-d Zone #3	OFF	5km walk Zone #1	OFF	Bohdan's Rhythm workout 2km w-up 2 x 100, 200, 300 w/ 100m Easy Walking between 1.5km c-d Zone #3 / #4	6km walk Zone #1	25km Total
8	3km walk Zone #1	Fartlek 2km w-up 4 x 400m/400m 1.5km c-d Make sure the kids don't start off too fast Zone #3 / #4	OFF	4km walk Zone #1	OFF	Bohdan's Rhythm workout 2km w-up 2 x 100, 200, 300 w/ 100m Easy Walking between 1.5km c-d Zone #3 / #4	6km walk Zone #1	25km Total
9	OFF	Speedwork 2km w-up 5 x 400m 2:00 rest 2km c-d Zone #3	3km walk Zone #1	OFF	2km easy walk	2km w-up 1-MILE RACE 1.5km c-d	5km walk Zone #1	20km Total
10	3km walk Zone #1	Team Relay races if you have enough teams. Pick your distance depending on how many kids there are.	OFF	5km walk Zone #1	OFF	Speedwork 1.5km w-up Fartlek 5 x 400m/400m 1.5km c-d Zone #3 / #4	6km walk Zone #1	30km Total
11	4km walk Zone #1	Fartlek 2km w-up 5 x 400/400m 1.5 km c-d Zone #3 / #4	OFF	5km walk Zone #1	OFF	2km w-up 2km Progression Walk 1.5km w-up EACH lap faster 5 seconds faster per lap	6km walk Zone #1	28km Total

Week	Monday	Tuesday	Wednesday	Thursday	Friday	Saturday	Sunday	Mileage
12	3km walk Zone #1	Fartlek 2km w-up 4 x 800m/400m 1.5 km c-d Zone #3	OFF	5km walk Zone #1	OFF	Bohdan's Rhythm workout 2km w-up 3 x 100, 200, 300 w/ 100m Easy Walking between 1.5km c-d Zone #3 / #4	6km walk Zone #1	29km Total
13	3km walk Zone #1	Fartlek 2km w-up 4 x 400/400m 1.5 km c-d Zone #3 / #4	OFF	5km walk Zone #1	OFF	Speedwork 2km w-up 1 x 800, 600, 400, 200m 3:00 rest 1.5km c-d Zone #3 / #4	5km walk Zone #1	25km Total
14	3km walk Zone #1	Speedwork 2km w-up 6 x 200m 2 min rest 1.5km c-d Zone #4	3km walk Zone #1	OFF	2km easy walk	Association Champs. 1-mile	3km easy walk	20km Total
15	4 km walk Zone #1	Speedwork 2 km w-up 5 x 400m 2 min rest 1.5km c-d Zone #4	OFF	5 km walk Zone #1	OFF	Bohdan's Rhythm workout 2km w-up 3 x 100, 200, 300 w/ 100m Easy Walking between 1.5km c-d Zone #4	6km walk Zone #1	26km Total

Phase IV - Peak Season for Youth Race Walkers

The Peak Season phase spans from week 16 through week 20 and is designed to prepare the athlete to walk his or her best race of the season at the Junior Olympics. "Best race" does not necessarily mean best time, as these championships take place in the hottest part of summer and are often scheduled in midday heat at a sweltering location. Since you can't control the start time or the weather, the goal of the race shouldn't be about pursuing a PR. The purpose of this training is to equip the young athlete to maximize effort throughout the race, including the last lap, of the last race of the season. Athletes should be reminded the conditions are the same for everyone on the track.

Week	Monday	Tuesday	Wednesday	Thursday	Friday	Saturday	Sunday	Mileage
16	3km walk Zone #1	Speedwork 1.5 km w-up 5 x 400m 2 min rest 1.5km c-d Zone #4	OFF	5km walk Zone #1	OFF	Bohdan's Rhythm workout 1.5km w-up 1 x 100, 200, 300 w/ 100m Easy Walking between 1.5km c-d Zone #4	3km walk Zone #1	21km Total
17	2km walk EASY	Regional Jr. Olympic Races	OFF	3km walk Zone #1	OFF	Speedwork 1.5km w-up 6 x 200m 1.5km c-d 2 min rest Zone #4	6km walk Zone #1	20km Total
18	3km walk Zone #1	Speedwork 1.5km w-up 1 x 800, 600, 400, 200 2:30 rest 1.5km c-d Zone #4	OFF	4km walk Zone #1	OFF	Speedwork 1.5km w-up 6 x 400m 1.5km c-d 2:30 rest Zone #4	5km walk Zone #1	22km Total
19	3km walk Zone #1	Speedwork 1.5km w-up 1 x 800, 600, 400, 200 2:30 rest 1.5km c-d Zone #4	OFF	4km walk Zone #1	OFF	Speedwork 1.5km w-up 3 x 400m 3 x 200m 2:30 rest 1.5km c-d Zone #4	4km walk Zone #1	21km Total
20	3km walk Zone #1	Speedwork 1.5km w-up 3 x 400m 1.5km c-d	3km walk Zone #1	OFF	2km walk Zone #1	Jr. Olympic Races		16km Total

A Few Essential Notes for Youth Race Walkers

About starting the race: The training has taught how fast an athlete can go for 1500 or 3000 meters. An athlete must not start faster than the prescribed speed, regardless of how fast the competition begins. It is very common for an excited young athlete to sprint the first 100 meters of a race and fade before the end of the first lap. Don't let this happen. Instead, maintain self-control so that there is energy and determination to fight when it counts—on the last lap.

About judges: It is easy for youth race walkers to view judges as the "bad guys," but they are there to ensure the competition is fair. If a judge shows an athlete a yellow paddle, they shouldn't slow down and crawl to the finish. Instead, they must refocus on proper technique. A paddle is just a warning, not necessarily a vote to disqualify an athlete. It takes three different judges to propose a disqualification for an athlete to be removed from the race.

About finishing the race: The last 100 meters call for special care. Many youths go all out at the end, especially if trying to edge out a competitor. When pushing hard it is easy to forget about proper form. So many times we have seen kids walk a perfect race and then get disqualified for running the last few meters. We want to celebrate after the race! Don't use that extra gear the last 20 meters, start your kick early.

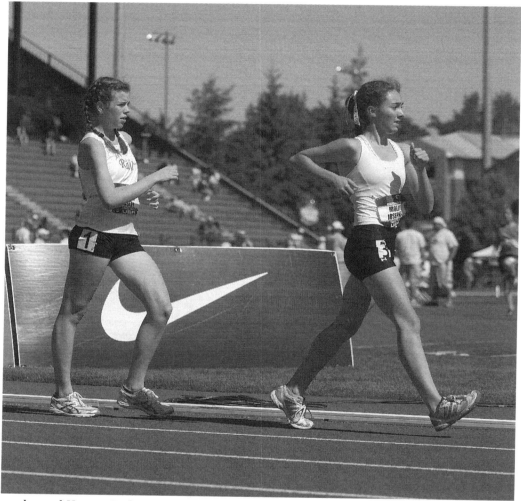

Molly Josephs and Hanna Kisley working together at the 2009 U.S. 10K Junior Nationals. Josephs got her start in the New York high school system and currently competes for Walk U.S.A. Kisley got started in the Junior Olympic program and currently competes for the Raleigh Walkers.

Chapter Five: Race Walking in High School

Both Jeff Salvage and I started race walking as high school athletes as part of the New York State high school program. At that time New York recognized race walking as a high school event for both boys and girls (now it is recognized only for girls, leaving Maine as the one state that offers high school race walking for both genders). As a result, our coaches trained us to walk the distance recognized in high school—one mile—as fast as possible. This approach becomes problematic when one considers all the significant opportunities available to a race walker—such as international competitions and college scholarships— which require walking longer distances.

Training and racing a mile is fun, but it's not ideal in the long term development for a race walker. This is not to say that competing at the one-mile distance is a mistake. The National Scholastic Indoor Championships, the Nike Indoor Nationals, and the New Balance Nationals offer the kids an incredible opportunity to compete in three track and field meets all of which have a rich, historic tradition. The National Scholastic Sports Foundation (NSSF), owners of the Nike Indoor and the New Balance Outdoor track and field meets, has been the driving force behind high quality high school race walking for both genders since its inception in 1990. Even prior to the formation of the NSSF, Tracy Sundlun, Mike Byrnes, and Jim Spier along with the Metropolitan Athletic Congress, supported race walking with the founding of the National Scholastic Indoor Championships in 1984. Competing in these events should be encouraged, but the focus of training should not be on peaking for them. Instead, athletes should race these championships as a milestone with a chance to earn All-American status and the opportunity to bring home a snazzy National Championship ring! What could motivate kids to try race walking more than to see their teammate strolling down the hallway with a super bowl-like ring around his/her finger? Another great race is the infamous Millrose Games, which includes a 1-mile walk. Many athletes have raced and performed well at the Games, while training for the 10km.

Even though there aren't as many walking scholarships as there are for running, one can find many lucrative opportunities. One South Texas Walking Club family is receiving $250,000 in free education for their two sons. The thanks go to race walking and Coach Jaime. Would you like to help your kids receive a scholarship? Get them race walking!

There are many opportunities to race walk at the international level. These opportunities include:

- World Race Walking Cup (10km Junior races for boys and girls)
- World Youth Track and Field Championships (10km boys and 5km girls)
- Junior Pan American Track and Field Championships (10km boys and girls)
- World Junior Track and Field Championships (10km boys and girls)
- Youth Olympic Games (10km boys and 5km girls)

To qualify for and excel at these international events, an athlete must train for more than just a one-mile race. The focus must be to train for the internationally accepted distances of 5km and 10km.

As the needs of high school race walkers vary greatly based upon their age and ability, we separate our advice for high school race walkers into two sections: grades 9-10 (ages 14-16) or for those who are just beginning to race walk and grades 11-12 (ages 16-18) or for those who have walked for a few years. Please note that just because someone is of a certain age, doesn't mean they should be forced to follow a more advanced level of training. The schedule and each workout must be based on a person's individual level of ability to maximize results. For all of these athletes we assume they already know how to race walk and we are detailing the training component of their routine. For those athletes still learning the basic technique, they must remember the technical component is more important than training fast. Please consult *Race Walk Clinic - in a Book* for information on the technique components of race walking.

Developing a Schedule for Early High School Race Walkers (Grades 9-10)

Most kids discover their favorite sport before high school, but I didn't start race walking until 11th grade and Jeff began as a high school senior. Neither of us knew it was an Olympic event when we started; we just knew our coach wanted us to walk a mile as fast as we could so that our teams could earn more points in dual meets. So instead of focusing on technique we focused on going really fast. As a result, it took me a long time to master the technique and to build a solid endurance base. This hampered my ability to improve in the long term. This focus on speed stayed with me through my first year of college. While I was highly successful that year, breaking four national junior records, it was not without a cost. The 18 months following my freshman year in college were wasted due to an injury I attribute to my limited endurance base.

The key to any successful walker is consistency of training, a theme we constantly reinforce throughout this book. Consistency comes from building a solid foundation of correct technique and an endurance base which should eliminate bad habits before they become embedded. Following this formula helps young athletes remain injury-free and is crucial for their short-term and long-term success. Injuries cause athletes to perform below their potential, get discouraged, and quit. Sadly, we have had many such examples in U.S. race walking; two recent ones were Lisa Kutzing and Katy Hayes, both of whom walked the mile around 7:00 in high school but who eventually quit due to injuries. While no training prescription can guarantee protection from injuries, the TEAMS method of training simply reduces their likelihood.

We focus on preparing the young high school walkers to race well at a one-mile, 3km or 5km event, while still having the ability to walk a few 10km races a year if they are strong enough. We have not placed 3km and 5km races on the schedule, other than the 3km Junior Olympic Championships, because there are so few available. However, you will have to place some races into the schedule depending upon when your association and regional qualifying events occur. Trying to include a specific local race on the schedule is difficult since everyone's local races occur at different times. Therefore, with the knowledge presented here, you should be able to adjust the sample schedule so that you don't go into the race tired, sore and risk an injury by following the sample taper schedules shown in chapter three.

Remember, no schedule is written in stone. If we could write the book's schedules in pencil, it would be preferable because you must be able to adapt the schedule to your own individual needs and life situations. It is much better to drop a workout than force it into a busy schedule where it doesn't fit. As you become familiar with the TEAMS philosophy of training you will be able to make these adjustments wisely for yourself or your athletes so that they can race walk faster by training smarter.

Setting the Schedule

Since the schedule is designed to be used any year, it is set up in a generic format based upon a typical young high school walker's schedule. We assume that most of the kids either run cross country in the fall, play soccer, or participate in some other sports. Therefore we started the first week of the season around November 1st and placed key races into the schedule approximately where they fall each year. Aspiring young elite walkers should consider competing at the National Scholastic Indoor Championships in the middle of March, the Penn Relays on the last Saturday in April, the USA Track and Field Junior Nationals in late June, or the Junior Olympic races near the end of July. These races give younger athletes goals and positive experiences with their peers. Each year builds upon the previous season so that you can get stronger and faster.

It is counterproductive to develop a full-year training schedule for high school walkers as we did for elite walkers. Younger athletes can't train for 50 weeks without their bodies breaking down. Also, as we discussed in chapter 4, you must keep workouts fresh and interesting, as 14- and 15-year-old athletes are still likely to get bored and move on to another sport if you aren't careful. We've even included some running workouts, since most youths come from some form of running background. Running is easier on the mind, because it does not require the constant focus on technique, and gives the body a break from any overuses caused by race walking. However, if you think running will cause injuries or other problems for an athlete, replace it with some other alternative activity.

This schedule has a five-week Early Season Base Work phase and then a four week Late Season Base Work phase. It is very difficult to keep a 14- or 15-year old focused for such a long period of time on "boring" base work, so we have kept it relatively short. We then return to the "early" phase in weeks 13 and 14 to allow the body to recover and prepare for a final push toward the National Scholastic races and Penn Relays. These modifications from a traditional elite schedule are done for psychological reasons as much as physiological ones.

Phase I - Early Season Base Work for Grades 9-10

The Early Season Base Work phase lasts just five weeks. The goal during this period is to allow the athlete's body to get accustomed to race walking again and to establish a foundation of endurance on which to build the remainder of the season. Technique drills and stretches must be part of the routine, so that you can work on nice, lean, flexible muscles. During these five weeks, no hard fartleks are performed. Instead, there are just a few days with pickups to keep the mind focused. Pickups are just workouts whereby you walk a little faster for the designated time. The pickups aren't done all out, they are just to get a good rhythm while focusing on good technique. Also, make sure the Zone #1 days are in fact walked in Zone #1. Don't push your workouts too fast. Instead, focus on building the engine. We will have plenty of time to fine-tune it later during the In Season Racing phase.

Week	Monday	Tuesday	Wednesday	Thursday	Friday	Saturday	Sunday	Mileage
1	3km walk Zone #1	4km easy run	4km walk Zone #1	OFF	4km easy run	4km walk Zone #1	45 min Hiking	23km Total
2	4km walk Zone #1	4km easy run	4km walk Zone #1	OFF	3km walk Zone #1	5km walk Zone #1	60 min Hiking	26km Total
3	5km walk Zone #1	5km easy run	5km walk Zone #1 w/ 4 x 1-min pickups after 2km	OFF	4km walk Zone #1	6km walk Zone #1	6km easy run	31 km total
4	6km walk with 5 x 1-min pickups after 2km	5km easy run	6km walk Zone #1	OFF	4km walk Zone #1	8km walk Zone #1	60 min Hiking	36km Total
5	6km walk Zone #1 with 5 x 2-min Pickups after 2km	5km easy run	7km walk Zone #1	OFF	5km walk Zone #1	8km walk Zone #1	60 min Hiking	38km Total

Phase II - Late Season Base Work for Grades 9-10

The Late Season Base Work phase lasts four weeks. It allows the body to adjust to doing one harder fartlek session per week, while also including longer workouts that do not put too much stress on the body. Many other programs introduce three hard days of repetitions per week at this point. This is a mistake. This is too soon to fine-tune an engine that isn't completely built. In other words, it is way too early to make large withdrawals from the bank. Don't push the body too hard—you don't want to miss weeks of training by getting injured. Remember, the key is consistency of training.

Week	Monday	Tuesday	Wednesday	Thursday	Friday	Saturday	Sunday	Mileage
6	5km walk Zone #1	Bohdan's Rhythm workout 2km w-up 3 x 100, 200, 300 with 100m easy walk between 2km c-d Zone #3	6km walk Zone #1	OFF	4km walk Zone #1	8km walk Zone #1	6km easy run	27 km Total
7	4km walk Zone #1	Fartlek 2km w-up 5 x 400/400m 2km c-d Zone #3	7km walk Zone #1	OFF	5km walk Zone #1	8km walk Zone #1	45 min Hiking	36 km Total

58

Week	Monday	Tuesday	Wednesday	Thursday	Friday	Saturday	Sunday	Mileage
8	Bohdan's Rhythm workout 2km w-up 3 x 100, 200, 300 w/ 100m easy walk between 2km c-d Zone #3 / #4	4km walk Zone #1	OFF	2km w-up 3 x 200 NO pushing 1km c-d Just get a good rhythm in your legs	15 min walk Zone #1	1-Mile race for Indoor Nationals qualifier or try to find some race to do	8km easy run	32km Total
9	OFF	5km walk Zone #1	5km run Zone #1	OFF	5km walk Zone #1	Fartlek 2km c-d 3 x 800/400m 2km c-d Zone #3	6km run Zone #1	32km Total

Phase III - In Season Racing for Grades 9-10

The In Season Racing phase lasts from week 10 through week 35. The goal is to get stronger, enter a few high quality races, and prepare the body and mind for the final peak phase. The In Season Racing phase allows the athlete to compete at a variety of distances, while still building the engine and depositing money into the bank. Coaches and athletes must take great care during this phase to react quickly to aches and pains to prevent them from becoming long-term injuries. Also, athletes must avoid exposure to activities that might increase their risk of getting sick and missing training time. Coaches should try to avoid placing stress on their athletes; high school is stressful enough for most of them.

The goal for young high school walkers in this phase is twofold: to walk a fast mile at one of the national one-mile indoor events as they prepare to compete in either a 5km for the girls, or a 10km for the boys, at the Penn Relays and to finish up this phase with a solid race at the USA Track and Field Junior Nationals in June. If a young athlete does not compete there, he or she should try to do a 3km or 5km race around the same time of year. During the time period between the Penn Relays and Junior Nationals, find a few races at distances of one mile to 5km to keep the training fresh. When doing so, use the taper and recovery sample schedules provided in chapter 3 to prepare for the race and then get back into the training program.

The following schedule for the In Season Racing phase is created for an ideal world. However, in high school programs like the one in New York State and Maine, the girls have numerous races throughout the season. Sometimes there are multiple races in one week. In this situation, following a taper for each race would be counterproductive. Some of the races, particularly those early season races, should be walked in place of one of the harder workouts for the week. They should not be tapered for, since they do not need to be peaked for, but care should be taken to make sure you are recovering properly.

Here is the In Season Racing phase:

Week	Monday	Tuesday	Wednesday	Thursday	Friday	Saturday	Sunday	Mileage
10	5km walk Zone #1	Fartlek 3km w-up 6 x 400/400 2km c-d is Zone #3/#4	8km walk Zone #1	OFF	5km walk Zone #1	Fartlek 3km w-up 1.2.3.3.2.1 min with equal Rest. 1 min fast, 1 min med, 2 min fast, 2 min med, etc. 2km c-d Zone #3	10km walk Zone #1	48km Total
11	6km walk Zone #1	Fartlek 2 km w-up 4 x 1km/500 2km c-d Zone #4	8km walk Zone #1	6km walk Zone #1	Bohdan's Rhythm workout 2km w-up 3 x 100, 200, 300, 400m w/ 100m easy between 2km c-d Zone #4	10km walk Zone #1	OFF, last day off to prepare for Milrose Games	48km total
12	Speedwork 2.5km w-up 3 x 500m 2 min rest 2km c-d Zone #3	4km walk Zone #1	4km walk Zone #1	3km easy walk with 3 x 100m pickups	1-mile RACE Millrose Games Or other 1-Mile or 3km race	75 min Hiking	8km to 10km walk Zone #1	43km Total
13 Rec. Week	OFF	6km walk Zone #1	8km walk Zone #1	6km easy run	5km walk Zone #1	12km walk Zone #1	OFF	37km Total
14 Rec. Week	6km walk Zone #1	10km walk Zone #1	6km walk Zone #1	10km walk Zone #1	OFF	12km walk Zone #1	8km easy run or walk Zone #1	56km Total

As noted above, weeks 13 and 14 are an intentional return to the Early Season Base Work phase. These two weeks allow the body to recover from the work done in weeks 1 through 12 as well as to prepare itself for the next phase of our season.

Week	Monday	Tuesday	Wednesday	Thursday	Friday	Saturday	Sunday	Mileage
15	6km walk Zone #1	Fartlek 2 km w-up 4 x 1km/500 2km c-d Zone #3	10km walk Zone #1	OFF	6-8km walk Zone #1	Progression walk 8km Each km is 5 sec faster per km. Zone #1 then Zone #2/ #3	12km walk Zone #1	60 km Total
16	6km walk Zone #1	Mexican speedwork 2km w-up 1 x 1000, 800, 600, 400, 200 2 min rest Zone # 3 or Zone # 4	10km walk Zone #1	OFF	8km walk Zone #1	Fartlek 2km w-up 4 x 1km/500m 2km c-d Zone # 3	12km walk Zone #1	53km total
17	6km walk Zone #1	Bohdan's Rhythm workout 2km w-up 3 x 100, 200, 300, 400 w/ 100m easy between 2km c-d Zone #4	6km walk Zone #1	OFF	5km walk Zone #1	2km w-up + pickups 1-MILE RACE Last chance qualifier for Indoor Nationals	8km walk Zone #1	39km Total
18	6km walk Zone #1	Mexican Speedwork 2km w-up 1 (or 2) x 1000, 800, 600, 400, 200 2km c-d Zone #3 / #4	8km walk Zone #1	OFF	6km walk Zone #1	Bohdan's Rhythm workout 3 x 100, 200, 300, 400m w/ 100m easy between 2km c-d Zone #4	8km walk Zone #1	46km total
19	4km walk Zone #1	Speedwork 2km w-up 6 x 400m 2 min rest 2 km c-d Zone #3	6km walk Zone #1	3km walk Zone #1 Or OFF	3km walk Zone #1	National Scholastic Indoor Champ. 1-mile RACE	Nike Indoor Nats. 1-Mile RACE	36km Total
20 Rec. Week	OFF	5km easy run	6km walk Zone #1	OFF	6km walk Zone #1	Fartlek 2km w-up 6 x 500/500 2km c-d Zone #3	12km walk Zone #1	39km Total

Week	Monday	Tuesday	Wednesday	Thursday	Friday	Saturday	Sunday	Mileage
21	6km walk Zone #1	Speedwork 2km w-up 2 (or 3) x 2km 3:00 rest 2km c-d Zone #2 / #3	8km walk Zone #1	OFF	5km easy run or walk Zone #1	Fartlek 2km w-up 4 x 1km/500m 2km c-d Zone # 3	12km walk Zone #1	54km total
22	6km walk Zone #1	Speedwork 2km w-up 3km, 2km, 1km 3:30 rest 2km c-d Zone #2 / #3	8km walk Zone #1	OFF	5km walk Zone #1	Fartlek 2km w-up 6 x 500/500 2km c-d Zone #3	12-15km walk Zone #1	54km Total
23	6km walk Zone #1	Speedwork 2km w-up 4 x 1600m 2km c-d Zone #3	8km walk Zone #1	OFF	5km run or walk	Fartlek 2km w-up 6 x 1km/500 2km c-d Zone #3	12km walk Zone #1	54km Total
24	6km walk Zone #1	Speedwork 2km w-up 3 (or 4) x 1600m 2km c-d Zone #3	6km walk Zone #1	OFF	5km walk Zone #1	Speedwork 2km w-up 5 x 1km 2:30-3:00 rest 2km c-d Zone #3	8km walk Zone #1	43km total
25	5km walk Zone #1	Speedwork 2km w-up 4 or 5 x 500m 2 min rest 2km c-d NO FASTER than your 10km pace	4km walk Zone #1	4km walk Zone #1	OFF	Penn Relays 10,000m for boys 5,000m for girls	6km easy run	41km Total
26 Rec. Week	OFF	5km easy run	6km walk Zone #1	OFF	8km walk Zone #1	12km walk Zone #1	OFF	31km Total
27	6km walk Zone #1	Speedwork 2km w-up 2km, 1500m, 1000m, 500m 3-4 min rest 2km c-d Zone # 3	10km walk Zone #1	OFF	6km walk Zone #1	Fartlek 2km w-up 5 x 1km/500m 2km c-d Zone # 3	10km walk Zone #1	53km Total
28	6km walk Zone #1	Speedwork 2km w-up 3 x 2km 3-4 min rest 2km c-d Zone # 3	10km walk Zone #1	OFF	6km easy run or walk Zone #1	Fartlek 2km w-up 5 x 1km/500m 2km c-d Zone #3	12km walk Zone #1	56km Total

Week	Monday	Tuesday	Wednesday	Thursday	Friday	Saturday	Sunday	Mileage
29	5km walk Zone #1	Fartlek 2km w-up 6 x 500/500 2km c-d Zone #3	10km walk Zone #1	OFF	8km walk Zone #1	Mexican Speedwork 2km w-up 2 x 1000, 800, 600, 400, 200 2 min rest 2km c-d Zone # 3 2nd set faster than the first	10km walk Zone #1	53km Total
30 Rec. Week	OFF	6km walk Zone #1	6km easy walk	OFF	8km walk Zone #1	12km walk Zone #1	6km easy run	40km Total
31	5km walk Zone #1	Speedwork 2km w-up 3 or 4 x 2km 2km c-d Zone #3	10km walk Zone #1	6km walk Zone #1	OFF	Speedwork 2km w-up 2 x 3km 5:00 rest 2km c-d Zone #3	12km walk Zone #1	53km total
32	6km walk Zone #1	Fartlek 2km w-up 6 x 500/500 2km c-d Zone #4	10km walk Zone #1	6km walk Zone #1	OFF	Speedwork 2km w-up 2km, 1500m, 1km, 500m 3:00 rest 2km c-d Zone #3	10km walk Zone #1	51km Total
33	6km walk Zone #1	Speedwork 2km w-up 5 x 1,000m 3:00 rest 2km c-d Zone #3	8km walk Zone #1	6km walk Zone #1	OFF	Speedwork 2km w-up 8 x 400m 2:00 rest 2km c-d Zone #4	6km walk Zone #1	44km total
34	5km walk Zone #1	Speedwork 2km w-up 5 x 500m 2km c-d 2 min rest Zone #3 No faster than 10km race pace	4km walk Zone #1	OFF Travel Day	3km walk Zone #1	USATF Junior National Championships 10,000m for both boys and girls ONLY for those qualified	OFF	31km Total

Phase IV - Peak Season for Grades 9-10

After week #35, the athlete enters the Peak Season phase. This phase prepares most younger high school race walkers to excel at the Junior Olympics, either USA Track and Field or AAU. Those in grades 9-10 who are strong enough to compete at Junior Nationals are learning how to compete at that distance; pursuing a high medal at Junior Olympics will usually be the primary focus.

At this point the athlete is preparing mentally and physically for the big day. Extra precautions must be taken to stay strong. If an extra day off or another easy day is required, take it. Consistency of training becomes especially important at this point. Sadly, toward the end of the season many coaches put too much stress on their younger athletes causing them to break down.

Here is the Peak Season phase:

Week	Monday	Tuesday	Wednesday	Thursday	Friday	Saturday	Sunday	Mileage
35	4km walk Zone #1	6km walk Zone #1	8km walk Zone #1	OFF	6km walk Zone #1	Fartlek 3km w-up 6 x 500/500m 2km c-d Zone #3	10km walk Zone #1	45 km Total
36	6km walk Zone #1	Speedwork 2km w-up 3 x 1000m 4 x 400m 2 min rest Zone #4 2km c-d	OFF	8km walk Zone #1	6km walk Zone #1	Mexican Speedwork 2km w-up 2 x 1000, 800, 600, 400, 200 2 min rest Zone #4	10km walk Zone #1	48km total
37	8km walk Zone #1	Speedwork 2km w-up 3 x 800m 4 x 400m 2 min rest 2km c-d Zone #4	OFF	8km walk Zone #1	6km walk Zone #1	Speedwork 2km c-d 2 x 500, 400, 300, 200, 100 2 min rest 2km c-d Zone #4	10km walk Zone #1	47km Total
38	6km walk Zone #1	Mexican Speedwork 2km w-up 2 x 1000, 800, 600, 400, 200 2 min rest Zone # 4	OFF	8km walk Zone #1	6km walk Zone #1	Bohdan's Rhythm workout 2km w-up 3 x 100, 200, 300, 400 2km c-d Zone #4	8km walk Zone #1	45 km Total
39	6km walk Zone #1	Speedwork 2km w-up 6 x 400m 2 min rest 2km c-d Zone #3	OFF	5km walk Zone #1	3km walk Zone #1	Jr. Olympic 3,000m Race		27 km total

Developing a Schedule for Later High School Race Walkers (Grades 11-12)

High school walkers in grades 11 and 12 train slightly different from their younger counterparts. If they are already experienced walkers, they continue to build their technical and endurance base while gradually shifting the focus from 5km to 10km distances. If the shift is sudden, it puts an athlete at a huge injury risk. As always, we must focus on range of motion exercises and stretching.

Older high school walkers' programs contain more daily/weekly mileage to prepare them to compete at the longer 10km distance. Training with more distance does not make a walker slower; instead it builds a more powerful engine so that when it is time to rev it up, a walker will be driving a Ferrari instead of a go-cart.

This additional training does not keep walkers from succeeding at the one-mile distance. It is far easier to focus on the internationally recognized race distance of 10km and step down to the mile than it is to try to step up from the mile to the 10km. Jeff Salvage tried the latter approach after having broken 7:00 in the mile in his first season. He then tried to walk a 10km with no base work under his belt. You can guess what happened. He walked a very fast first mile and, by comparison crawled the rest of the 10km. He finished with a less than stellar time of about 55 minutes. The next year he walked a 45:30 for 10km and around a 6:30 mile. How did he accomplish the transformation? By training for the 10km, not the mile. Clearly, his mile time did not suffer and neither will yours.

As a walker gets older, the most important races are longer: USA Track and Field Junior Nationals, Penn Relays, and, for the very elite, the World Youth Championships for ages 16-17; and the World Junior Track and Field Championships for ages 16-19 are all races of 5km or 10kms. While a huge amount of development can occur between ages 16 and 19, it does not mean that younger athletes can't compete with the best. Susana Feitor from Portugal, who won the first global title of her career when she was just 15 years of age, captured gold in the 1990 World Junior Championships 5,000m walk with a time of 21:44. A year later she qualified to compete in the 10km walk at the IAAF World Track and Field Championships, a pinnacle of athletic competition, second only to the Olympic Games. This was the first of her record ten appearances at the World Championships. A year after that, at just seventeen years of age, Susana qualified for the first of her five Olympics.

Susana Feitor's example shows you can train well at a young age and still have a very long and successful career. Susana was one of the best in the world for the past 19 years. Many coaches are afraid to push their younger athletes into doing "too much" distance because they are afraid their athletes will get hurt. Like everything in training it's about balance. The key isn't to push the workouts, the key is to train smart by balancing distance and effort from day to day and week to week. You cannot push the body day after day, but if you train smart you can have success over the long haul.

The following schedule is based on the timetable of a traditional high school student. Most students go to school at about 8am and get out about 3pm. Therefore, on weekdays there are no second workouts scheduled. Given the amount of time spent at school, it would be too stressful. However, on Saturday afternoons there is occasionally an extra workout scheduled to help you before the longer walk on Sunday. If you are home schooled or have a more flexible schedule, additional workouts can be added. Remember though, consistency is the key. If you walk a lot of mileage one week and the following week you get sick because you didn't recover enough, then the extra mileage accomplished nothing. For those who have the time to add to their training use the advanced high school schedule as a starting point and adjust it to fit.

Phase I - Early Season Base Work for Grades 11 and 12
As with younger high school walkers, the Early Season Base Work phase last five weeks. The main goal is to get the body accustomed to race walking again. We assume that most walkers are

transitioning from their cross-country season or another sport, so for the first few weeks we have included running to ease the transition.

If any significant aches and pains occur during the transition back to walking, as always, apply common sense and back off the schedule a bit. Technique drills and stretching must be done regularly and correctly, as they pay dividends later.

Week	Monday	Tuesday	Wednesday	Thursday	Friday	Saturday	Sunday	Mileage
1	3km walk Zone #1	6km easy run	4km walk Zone #1	OFF	6km easy run	4km walk Zone #1	45 min Hiking	27km Total
2	4km walk Zone #1	6km easy run	6km walk Zone #1	OFF	3km walk Zone #1	6km walk Zone #1	60 min Hiking	26km Total
3	5km walk Zone #1	5km easy run	6km walk Zone #1 w/ 4 x 1-min pickups	8km walk Zone #1	OFF	8km walk Zone #1	8km easy Run	40 km total
4	6km walk with 5 x 1-min pickups After 2km	6km easy run	8km walk Zone #1	6km walk Zone #1	OFF	10km walk Zone #1	10km Hiking	41km Total
5	6km walk Zone #1 with 5 x 2-min Pickups after 2km	8km easy run	8km walk Zone #1	6km walk Zone #1	OFF	10km walk Zone #1	10km Hiking	43km Total

Phase II - Late Season Base Work for Grades 11 and 12

The Late Season Base Work phase lasts eight weeks and culminates, for those who qualify, with the Millrose Games one-mile race. The goal of this phase is to get the body walking fast while not overly taxing it with too many hard sessions. There is still a long season ahead and we do not want to peak too early. While you do not want to peak for a mile race this early in the season, the Millrose Games is recommended as an electrifying goal to pursue, because there is nothing like the excitement of competing before 15,000 fans in New York's Madison Square Garden. Many high schools records were set on the infamous track and it is an internationally prominent meet that attracts numerous Olympians every year. If an athlete doesn't qualify, he/she needn't stress about it. Instead, substitute a race around the same time. It is important not to take too long a break between races.

This phase includes just one speedwork or fartlek session per week until week #10. Then, we add an additional harder day to prepare your body for your mile race. We also add some second workouts, typically an easy run or aqua jogging, to allow you to flush the lactic acid out of your legs and enable you to feel fresher the following day.

Week	Monday	Tuesday	Wednesday	Thursday	Friday	Saturday	Sunday	Mileage
6	5km walk Zone #1	Bohdan's Rhythm workout 2km w-up 3 x 100, 200, 300, 400 with 100m easy walk between 2km c-d Zone #4	8km walk Zone #1	OFF	5km walk Zone #1	10km walk Zone #1	8km easy run	44km Total
7	5km walk Zone #1	Fartlek 2km w-up 8 x 400/400m 2km c-d Zone #4	8km walk Zone #1	OFF	6km walk Zone #1	8km walk Zone #1	10km Hiking	49km Total
8	Bohdan's Rhythm workout 2km w-up 3 x 100, 200, 300 w/100m easy walk between 2km c-d Zone #4	4km walk Zone #1	OFF	2km w-up 3 x 200 NO pushing 1km c-d Just get a good rhythm in your legs	15 min easy walk	1-Mile race to qualify for National Scholastic Indoor Championships or Millrose Games	6km easy run	30km Total
9	OFF	5km easy run	10km walk Zone #1	6km walk Zone #1	6km walk Zone #1	Fartlek 2km w-up 3 x 2km/1km 2km c-d Zone #2 DO NOT push these too much!	12km walk Zone #1	52km Total
10	5km walk Zone #1	Fartlek 2km w-up 10 x 400/400 2km c-d Zone #4	8km walk Zone #1	OFF	8km easy run	Fartlek 2km w-up 6 x 800/400 2km c-d Zone #3 -------------- 5km easy run	12km walk Zone #1	60km Total

Week	Monday	Tuesday	Wednesday	Thursday	Friday	Saturday	Sunday	Mileage
11	6km walk Zone #1	Fartlek 2.5 km w-up 5 x 1km/500 2km c-d Zone # 3	8km walk Zone #1	6km walk Zone #1	Bohdan's Rhythm workout 2km w-up 3 x 100, 200, 300, 400m w/ 100m Easy Between 2km c-d Zone #4	10km walk Zone #1	OFF	50km Total
12	Speedwork 3km w-up 4 x 500m 2 min rest 2km c-d Zone #3/#4	5km walk Zone #1	4km walk Zone #1 or OFF	3km easy walk with 3 x 100m pickups	Millrose Games 1-mile race Or Other 1-Mile or 3km race	10km Hiking	12km walk Zone #1	47km Total
13	OFF	8km walk Zone #1	8km walk Zone #1	6km easy run	5km walk Zone #1	Fartlek 3km w-up 8 x 500/500m 2km c-d Zone #3 — — — — — 5km easy run	12km walk Zone #1	57 km Total

Phase III - In Season Racing for Grades 11 and 12

The In Season Racing phase begins after week 13 and continues through week 34. This phase lasts for a long time, and it can be tough to stay focused. Therefore, it is important to find some competitions to break up the routine. The two one-mile indoor races in March, the Penn Relays in April, and the trials race for, depending on the year, either the World Race Walking Cup or America's Cup, are good options. The trials races are not included on the sample schedule because the date varies greatly, but they offer high-level competition and an opportunity to meet the time standard for the Penn Relays, as well as to qualify for the USATF Junior Nationals or even the World Junior Track and Field Championships or World Youth Track and Field Championships.

It is also important to give high school athletes recovery weeks, especially after races, to enable the body to absorb the preceding weeks of hard training and allow deposits in the body bank to accrue interest. If you are entering other competitions during this phase, just follow the templates for tapering and recovering shown in chapter 3. This will give you the best opportunity to feel fresh on race day, and as Olympic Champion Robert Korzeniowski taught me, don't "carry" the competition beyond the race course. He meant it is very important for you to recover as quickly as possible so that your body can focus on the future.

Week	Monday	Tuesday	Wednesday	Thursday	Friday	Saturday	Sunday	Mileage
14	6km walk Zone #1	Fartlek 3km w-up 5 x 1km/500m 2km c-d Zone #3	12km walk Zone #1	OFF	10km walk Zone #1	Bohdan's Rhythm workout 3km w-up 4 x 100, 200, 300, 400 w/ 100m easy between 2km c-d Zone #4 5km easy run	12km walk Zone #1	61km Total
15	6km walk Zone #1	Fartlek 2.5 km w-up 8 x 500m/500m 2km c-d Zone #3	10km walk Zone #1	OFF	6-8km walk Zone #1	Progression walk 2km w-up 6km 2km c-d Each km is 10 sec faster per km. Don't start off too fast! Zone #2 / #3 5km easy run	15km walk Zone #1	67km Total
16	6km walk EASY	Mexican Speedwork 2km w-up 2 x 1000, 800, 600, 400, 200 Zone #3 / #4 2 min rest	10km walk Zone #1	OFF	8km walk Zone #1	Fartlek 2km w-up 6 x 1km/500m 2km c-d Zone # 3 6km easy run	12km walk Zone #1	66km total
17	6km walk Zone #1	Bohdan's Rhythm workout 2km w-up 4 x 100, 200, 300, 400 w/ 100m easy between 2km c-d Zone #4	8km walk Zone #1	OFF	6km walk Zone #1	Mexican Speedwork 2km w-up 2 x 1000, 800, 600, 400, 200 2km c-d 2:00 rest Zone # 3/# 4 4km easy run	15km walk Zone #1	57km Total
18	6km walk Zone #1	Speedwork 2km w-up 5 x 1km 5 x 200m 2:30 rest 2km c-d Zone #3 / #4	10km walk Zone #1	OFF	8km walk Zone #1	Bohdan's Rythm workout 2km w-up 3 x 100, 200, 300, 400m w/ 100m easy between 2km c-d Zone #4	8km walk Zone #1	50km total

Week	Monday	Tuesday	Wednesday	Thursday	Friday	Saturday	Sunday	Mileage
19	4km walk Zone #1	Speedwork 2km w-up 6 x 400m @ + 10 sec/mile of goal pace	6km walk Zone #1	4km walk Zone #1 Or OFF	4km walk Zone #1	Nike Indoor Nationals 1-Mile Race	National Scholastic Indoor Nationals 1-Mile race	36km Total
20	OFF	5km easy run	6km walk Zone #1	OFF	6km walk Zone #1	Fartlek 2km w-up 8 x 500/500 2km c-d Zone #3	15km walk Zone #1	44km Total
21	6km walk Zone #1	Fartlek 2km w-up 5 x 1km/500m 2km c-d Zone #3	8km walk Zone #1	OFF	5km easy run or walk Zone #1	Fartlek 2km w-up 3 x 2km/1km 2km c-d Zone # 3 / 4km easy run	14km walk Zone #1	60km Total
22	6km walk Zone #1	Speedwork 2km w-up 3km, 2km, 1km, then 2 x 500m 3:30 rest 2km c-d Zone # 3	10km walk Zone #1	OFF	5km walk Zone #1	Fartlek 2km w-up 8 x 500/500 2km c-d Zone # 3 / 5km easy run	15km walk Zone #1	65km Total
23	6km walk Zone #1	Fartlek 2km w-up 4 x 1600m/800m 2km c-d Zone # 3	10km walk Zone #1	OFF	5km easy run or walk Zone #1	Fartlek 2km w-up 6 x 1km/500 2km c-d Zone # 3 / 6km easy run	15km walk Zone #1	65km Total
24	6km walk Zone #1	Speedwork 2km w-up 4 x 1600m 2km c-d 3:00 rest Zone # 3	8km walk Zone #1	OFF	6km walk Zone #1	Speedwork 2km w-up 6 x 1km Zone # 3 2km c-d 2:30 rest	8km walk Zone #1	48km total
25	5km walk Zone #1	Speedwork 2km w-up 6 x 500m 2 min rest 2km c-d NO FASTER than your 10km pace	5km walk Zone #1	4km walk Zone #1	OFF	Penn Relays 10,000m race for Boys 5,000m for girls	6km Run	41km Total
26 Rec. Week	OFF	5km easy run	6km walk Zone #1	OFF	8km walk Zone #1	12km walk Zone #1	OFF	31km Total

Week	Monday	Tuesday	Wednesday	Thursday	Friday	Saturday	Sunday	Mileage
27	6km walk Zone #1	Speedwork 2km w-up 2km, 1500m, 1000m, 500m 3-4 min rest 2km c-d Zone #3	10km walk Zone #1	OFF	6km walk Zone #1	Fartlek 2km w-up 6 x 1km/500m 2km c-d Zone #3	12km to 15km walk Zone #1	60km Total
28	6km walk Zone #1	Fartlek 2km w-up 3 x 2km/1km 2km c-d Zone #3	10km walk Zone #1	OFF	6km easy run or walk Zone #1	Fartlek 2km w-up 6 x 1km/500m 2km c-d Zone #3 4km easy run	15km walk Zone #1	63km Total
29	OFF	8km walk Zone #1	6km walk Zone #1	OFF	8km walk Zone #1	Speedwork 2km w-up 8 x 1km 2km c-d 2 min rest Zone #3	10km walk Zone #1	44km Total
30	5km walk Zone #1	TEMPO 2km w-up 6km Zone # 2 2km c-d	10km walk Zone #1	OFF	8km walk Zone #1	Mexican Speedwork 2km w-up 2 x 1000, 800, 600, 400, 200 2 min rest 2km c-d Zone #3 / #4 2nd set faster than the first	15km walk Zone #1	58km Total
31	6km walk Zone #1	Fartlek 2km w-up 3 x 2km/1km 2km c-d Zone #3	10km walk Zone #1	OFF	6km easy walk	Fartlek 2km w-up 5 x 1km/500 2km c-d Zone #3	15km walk Zone #1	60km Total
32	6km walk Zone #1	Fartlek 2km w-up 6 or 8 x 500/500 2km c-d Zone #3	10km walk Zone #1	OFF	6km walk Zone #1	Speedwork 2km w-up 2 x 3km 4:00 rest 2km c-d Zone #2 / #3 These are done at your 10km pace, no faster	15km walk Zone #1	55km Total
33	6km walk Zone #1	Speedwork 2km w-up 4 x 1600m 2:30 rest 2km c-d Zone #3	8km walk Zone #1	OFF	6km walk Zone #1	Speedwork 2km w-up 6 x 1km 2:30 rest 2km c-d Zone #3	6km walk Zone #1	45km total

Week	Monday	Tuesday	Wednesday	Thursday	Friday	Saturday	Sunday	Mileage
34	5km walk Zone #1	Speedwork 2km w-up 5 x 500m 2km c-d 2 min rest No faster than goal pace	4km walk Zone #1	OFF Travel Day	3km walk Zone #1	USATF Junior National Championships 10,000m for both boys and girls	OFF	31km Total

Phase IV - Peak Season Grades 11 and 12

The Peak Season phase lasts from week 35 through 39. School is out and there is much more time to train, but this does not mean you should force more mileage into the schedule. It is the solid recovery from the harder days that is the key to better performances. The sole focus of this phase is to peak for your most important race, which might be a major international competition, the USA vs. Canada dual meet, the Junior Olympics, or perhaps an open race in your state, such as the Empire State Games in New York or the Keystone Games in Pennsylvania. Stay consistent with the training and stay focused on technique as more speed is added to the program. You do not want to end your season with a disqualification, so good, efficient technique must always be stressed.

Week	Monday	Tuesday	Wednesday	Thursday	Friday	Saturday	Sunday	Mileage
35	4km walk Zone #1	6km walk Zone #1	OFF	8km walk Zone #1	6km walk Zone #1	Fartlek 3km w-up 8 x 500m/500m 2km c-d Zone #3	12km walk Zone #1	49km Total
36	6km walk Zone #1	Speedwork 2km w-up 6 x 1000m 5 x 400m 2 min rest Zone #4 2km c-d	10km walk Zone #1	OFF	6km walk Zone #1	Mexican Speedwork 2km w-up 2 x 1000, 800, 600, 400, 200 2 min rest Zone #4 6km run	12km walk Zone #1	62km total
37	8km walk Zone #1	Speedwork 2km w-up 6 x 800m 6 x 400m 2 min rest 2km c-d Zone #4	8km walk Zone #1	OFF	6km walk Zone #1	Speedwork 2km c-d 3 x 500, 400, 300, 200, 100 2 min rest 2km c-d Zone #4 5km run	15km walk Zone #1	62km Total
38	8km walk Zone #1	Mexican Speedwork 2km w-up 2 x 1000, 800, 600, 400, 200 2 min rest Zone #4	8km walk Zone #1	OFF	6km walk Zone #1	Bohdan's Rhythm workout 2km w-up 4 x 100, 200, 300, 400 2km c-d	10km walk Zone #1	51km Total
39	6km walk Zone #1	Speedwork 2km w-up 6 x 400m 2km c-d Zone #3	5km walk Zone #1	OFF	3km walk Zone #1	Jr. Olympic 3,000m Race or USA vs Canada Dual meet 10km or 5km		33km total

Developing a Schedule for Elite High School Race Walkers

Elite race walkers are a different breed. Walkers in high school who strive to walk at an elite level follow a different training program than their peers. Their schedule starts earlier, giving them more time to prepare for their peak season. Our schedule assumes that an athlete will not be running cross country. It does not mean though that you must skip cross country to be an elite level race walker. There are actually benefits to having a running season. This is especially true of beginning walkers who are still trying to get stronger and learn the proper time to push in a race. If your athlete falls into this category, they should train using the previous training schedule instead of this one. In contrast, solid competitors who have already walked some pretty fast times and have trained their bodies to handle the stress of distance and intensity are the type of walkers we are targeting with this schedule.

Phase I - Early Season Base Work for Elite High School Walkers:

The Early Season Base Work phase for the elite high school athlete begins around October 1st. It lasts nine weeks and the goal is to get the athlete strong enough to handle the rest of the season.

Week	Monday	Tuesday	Wednesday	Thursday	Friday	Saturday	Sunday	Mileage
1	5km walk Zone #1	6km easy run	6km walk Zone #1	OFF	8km easy run	6km walk Zone #1	8km Hiking	39km Total
2	10km walk Zone #1	8km easy run	8km walk Zone #1	OFF	10km walk Zone #1	10km walk Zone #1	10km Hiking	56km Total
3	10km walk Zone #1	10km easy run	10km walk Zone #1	OFF	8km walk Zone #1	12km walk Zone #1	12km Hiking	62km total
4	8km walk Zone #1	10km easy run	12km walk Zone #1	OFF	10km walk Zone #1 / 5km easy run	15km walk Zone #1	15km Hiking	75km Total
5	8km walk Zone #1	10km easy run	12km walk Zone #1	OFF	10km walk Zone #1 / 5km easy run	15km walk Zone #1	18km Hiking	78km Total
6	8km walk Zone #1	2km w-up LACTATE TEST 6 x 2km 2km c-d	15km walk Zone #1	12km walk Zone #1	6km easy run	18km walk Zone #1	15km Hiking	90km Total
7	10km walk Zone #1 / 6km easy run	10km Progression walk Zone #1 then Zone #2 / #3	15km walk Zone #1	12km walk Zone #1	6km easy run	18km walk Zone #1	15km Hiking	92km Total

Week	Monday	Tuesday	Wednesday	Thursday	Friday	Saturday	Sunday	Mileage
8	10km walk Zone #1 6km easy run	10km walk Zone #1	15km walk Zone #1	12km walk Zone #1 4km easy run	8km walk Zone #1	12km Progression Walk Zone #1 then Zone #2 / #3 5km easy run	18km walk Zone #1	100km Total
9 Rec. Week	8km walk Zone #1 4km run	OFF	12km walk Zone #1	8km walk Zone #1	OFF	10km easy run	15km walk Zone #1	57km Total

Phase II - Late Season Base Work for Elite High School Walkers:

The elite high school walker trains very differently during the Late Season Base Work phase than the traditional high school race walker. Their mileage is higher and they walk with more intensity. The goal of this phase is to begin working on upper end speed with shorter fartleks while also working on strength with longer fartleks. Please notice the holidays built into the schedule. Christmas Day, Christmas Eve, New Years Day and New Years Eve are all there. Since we are starting this schedule around October 1st, they fall during weeks 13 and 14. During the course of my career it was very frustrating for me to see very hard workouts on those days and it was also extremely irritating for my family who needed my help during that time. Therefore, during these days taking a day OFF or walking an easier workout can reduce stress. One stressful year my coach required me to walk an incredulous 30 miles on Christmas Eve. In the freezing cold, Will Van Axen and I braved the temperatures and finished our trek across Long Island. The next week I was sick and missed almost the whole week due to illness. Don't let this happen to you, be smart during this time. The holidays are stressful enough.

Week	Monday	Tuesday	Wednesday	Thursday	Friday	Saturday	Sunday	Mileage
10	12km walk Zone #1 8km easy run	Fartlek Bohdan's Rhythm Workout 5km easy run	15km walk Zone #1	12km walk Zone #1	8km walk Zone #1	Fartlek 3km w-up 2 x 4km/1km Zone # 2 2km c-d	18km walk Zone #1	105km Total
11	12km walk Zone #1	Fartlek Bohdan's Rhythm Workout 6km easy run	15km walk Zone #1	12km walk Zone #1 6km easy run	10km walk Zone #1	Fartlek 3km w-up 2 x 5km /1km Zone # 2 2km c-d 6km easy run	12km walk Zone #1	107km Total
12	18km walk Zone #1	12km walk Zone #1 6km easy run	15km walk Zone #1	8km easy run Christmas Eve	Christmas DAY OFF	Fartlek 3km w-up 3 x 3km/1km ZONE # 2 2km c-d 6km easy run	18km walk Zone #1	100km Total

Week	Monday	Tuesday	Wednesday	Thursday	Friday	Saturday	Sunday	Mileage
13	12km walk Zone #1	Speedwork 2km w-up 10 x 500m 2 min rest 2km c-d	10km walk Zone #1	New Years Eve 10km walk Zone #1	New Years Day 8km easy run	6km walk Zone #1	3,000m Indoor Qualifying race	63km Total
14 Rec. Week	6km walk Zone #1	12km walk Zone #1	15km walk Zone #1	OFF	10km walk Zone #1	Fartlek 3km w-up 2 x 4km /1km Zone # 2 2km c-d 6km easy run	18km walk Zone #1	82km Total
15	12km walk Zone #1	14km walk Zone #1 6km easy run	18km walk Zone #1	12km walk Zone #1	12km walk Zone #1	Fartlek 3km w-up 2 x 6km/1km Zone # 2 2km c-d	18km walk Zone #1	110km Total
16	12km walk Zone #1	Mexican Speedwork 3km w-up 3 x 1000, 800, 600, 400, 200 2km c-d Zone # 4 5km easy run	15km walk Zone #1	12km walk Zone #1	Bohdan's Rhythm workout 3km w-up 4 x 100, 200, 300, 400 w/ 100m easy between 2km c-d Zone # 4 6km easy run	18km walk Zone #1	12km walk Zone #1	105km Total
17	Speedwork 3km w-up 10 x 500m 90 second rest 2km c-d 5km easy run	15km walk Zone #1	12km walk Zone #1	8km walk Zone #1	3km Pedestrian Walk - AM Millrose Games 1-Mile RACE	12km walk Zone #1	20km walk Zone #1	90km Total

Phase III - In Season Racing for Elite High School Walkers:

The In Season Racing phase lasts from week #18 through week # 38. Care must be taken to make sure you maintain your range of motion and flexibility by stretching and performing mobility exercises and technique drills. While stretching should be performed after every workout, if you are limited on time, try to do at least a few techniques drills every day. At least two to three days a week do the complete set.

This phase includes the USATF Indoor Nationals, the two high school Indoor Scholastic Championships, as well as either the World Cup or America's Cup Trials on the weekend that it is typically held. **We purposely did not put these events onto the schedule because they vary greatly upon which weekend they occur. Instead for now, we have placed training where those races may occur. When you know the exact dates of the race adjust the schedule as per a typical taper week and recover week that we have shown in chapter 3.**

You should be able to adjust almost any two weeks (one for the taper and race, and the other for the recovery week) from this phase and still build your engine.

Week	Monday	Tuesday	Wednesday	Thursday	Friday	Saturday	Sunday	Mileage
18	OFF	Fartlek 3km w-up 10 x 500/500 2km c-d Zone #3 / 6km easy run	12km walk Zone #1	12km walk Zone #1	10km walk Zone #1	3km w-up Norwegian Fartlek 2km c-d Zone #3 / 6km easy run	15km walk Zone #1	91km Total
19	8km walk Zone #1	2km w-up LACTATE TEST 6 x 2km 2km c-d / 6km easy run	15km walk Zone #1	OFF	10km walk Zone #1	Fartlek 2km w-up 8 x 1km/500m 2km c-d Zone #3 / 6km easy run	20km walk Zone #1	97km Total
20	8km walk Zone #1	Speedwork 3km w-up 3 x 4km 2:30 rest 2km c-d Zone # 2/ #3 / 4km easy run	16km walk Zone #1	12km walk Zone #1 / 6km easy run	10km walk Zone #1	Fartlek 3km w-up 8 x 1km/500m 2km c-d Zone # 3 / 6km easy run	20km walk Zone #1	116km Total
21	8km walk Zone #1	Speedwork 3km w-up 5 x 2km 2:00 rest 2km c-d Zone # 3 / 6km easy run	18km walk Zone #1	12km walk Zone #1 / 6km easy run	12km walk Zone #1	Mexican Speedwork 3km w-up 3 x 1000, 800, 600, 400, 200 2km c-d 2 min rest Zone # 4 / 6km easy run	20km walk Zone #1	117km Total

Week	Monday	Tuesday	Wednesday	Thursday	Friday	Saturday	Sunday	Mileage
22	10km walk Zone #1	Fartlek 3km w-up 12 x 500/500 2km c-d Zone #3 / #4 5km easy run	15km walk Zone #1	OFF	12km walk Zone #1	Speedwork 3km w-up 10 x 1km 2 min rest 2km c-d Zone # 3	12km walk Zone #1	86km Total
23	12km walk Zone #1	Speedwork 3km w-up 12 x 500m 90 sec rest 2km c-d Zone # 3	12km walk Zone #1	8km walk Zone #1	6km walk Zone #1	USATF Indoor Nationals 5,000m for men 3,000m for women	12km walk Zone #1	71km Total
24 Rec. Week	16km walk Zone #1	10km walk Zone #1 5km easy run	OFF	15km walk Zone #1	12km walk Zone #1	Bohdan's Rhythm workout 3km w-up 4 x 100, 200, 300, 400m with 100m easy between 2km c-d Zone # 4 6km easy run	15km walk Zone #1	90km Total
25	8km walk Zone #1	Speedwork 3km w-up 5 x 1km 6 x 500m 2 min rest 2km c-d Zone # 3	15km walk Zone #1	12km walk Zone #1	6km walk Zone #1	Nike Indoor Nationals 1-Mile Race	National Scholastic Indoor Championships 1-Mile Race	64km Total
26	6km easy run	OFF	12km walk Zone #1	12km walk Zone #1 6km easy run	8km walk Zone #1	Speedwork 3km w-up 5 x 2km 2 min rest 2km c-d Zone #3 6km easy run	15km walk Zone #1	80km Total
27	12km walk Zone #1	3km w-up 10 x 500 m 2km c-d Zone #4 5km easy run	12km walk Zone #1	10km walk Zone #1	6km walk Zone #1	10km RACE (World Cup Trials or America's Cup Trials)	8km easy run	78km Total
28 Rec. Week	OFF	12km walk Zone #1	18km walk Zone #1	OFF	12km walk Zone #1	Fartlek 3km w-up 12 x 500/500 2km c-d Zone #3	20km walk Zone #1	79km Total

Week	Monday	Tuesday	Wednesday	Thursday	Friday	Saturday	Sunday	Mileage
29	12km walk Zone #1	Speedwork 3km w-up 6 x 2km 2 min rest 2km c-d Zone #3 / 6km easy run	18km walk Zone #1	12km walk Zone #1	8km walk Zone #1	Speedwork 3km w-up 10 x 1km 2 min rest 2km c-d Zone #3 / 6km easy run	15km walk Zone #1	103km Total
30	10km walk Zone #1	Speedwork 3km w-up 10 x 500m 2 min rest 2km c-d Zone #3	12km walk Zone #1	8km walk Zone #1	6km walk Zone #1	Penn Relays 10,000m boys 5,000m girls	15km walk Zone #1	75km Total
31	12km walk Zone #1	12km walk Zone #1 / 5km easy run	18km walk Zone #1	OFF	10km walk Zone #1	Fartlek 3km w-up 3 x 4km/1km 2km c-d Zone #2 / #3	18km walk Zone #1	95km Total
32	12km walk Zone #1	Fartlek 3km w-up 8 x 1km/500 2km c-d Zone #3 / 5km easy run	15km walk Zone #1	8km walk Zone #1	12km walk Zone #1	Fartlek 3km w-up 5 x 2km/1km 2km c-d Zone #3 / 4km easy run	18km walk Zone #1	111km Total
33 Rec. Week	OFF	12km walk Zone #1	15km walk Zone #1	12km walk Zone #1	12km walk Zone #1	Fartlek 3km w-up 12 x 500/500 2km c-d Zone #3	18km walk Zone #1	86km Total
34	8km walk Zone #1	Speedwork 3km w-up 3 x 2km 4 x 1km 2km c-d 2 min rest Zone #2 / #3 / 6km easy run	15km walk Zone #1	12km walk Zone #1	10km walk Zone #1	TEMPO 3km w-up 8km walk Zone #2 2km c-d / 6km easy run	15km walk Zone #1	100km Total
35	12km walk Zone #1	Fartlek 3km w-up 3 x 4km/1km 2km c-d Zone #3 / 5km easy run	15km walk Zone #1	12km walk Zone #1 / 6km easy run	10km walk Zone #1	Fartlek 3km w-up 10 x 1km/500 2km c-d Zone #3	18km walk Zone #1	118km Total

Week	Monday	Tuesday	Wednesday	Thursday	Friday	Saturday	Sunday	Mileage
36	10km walk Zone #1	Speedwork 3km w-up 6 x 2km 2km c-d Zone #3 / 6km easy run	18km walk Zone #1	12km walk Zone #1 / 6km easy run	10km walk Zone #1	Speedwork 3km w-up 4 x 3km 2km c-d Zone #3 / 6km easy run	18km walk Zone #1	120km Total
37	12km walk Zone #1	Speedwork 3km w-up 6 x 2km 2km c-d Zone #3 / 4km run	15km walk Zone #1	12km walk Zone #1	12km walk Zone #1	Speedwork 3km w-up 10 x 1km 2 min rest 2km c-d Zone #3 / 4km run	12km walk Zone #1	103km Total
38	12km walk Zone #1	3km w-up Norwegian Fartlek 2km c-d	12km walk Zone #1	8km walk Zone #1 with pickups	6km walk Zone #1	USATF Jr. National Championships	8km easy run	74km Total

Phase IV - Peak Season for Elite High School Walkers:

As an athlete or coach, the Peak Season phase is one of the hardest aspects of training to perfect. On week #40 of the 2009 season, both Rachel Lavallee, now Rachel Seaman, and Trevor Barron raced the best competitions of their lives at their biggest international events. They competed in two very different competitions. Rachel walked in the World University Games, while Trevor participated in the World Youth Track and Field Championships. The peak phase presented is similar to the one Trevor followed during his successful season. Trevor raced twice during his peak phase. First, he walked a 42:22 to set the U.S. Junior National record at the World Youth Championships while placing fourth. A few short weeks later he raced again. The second race was slower, but it was tactically a much smarter race and under the tough Caribbean conditions on the small island of Trinidad and Tobago. He placed 4th as a 16 year old, walking 42:50.

Racing and traveling internationally almost always poses some sort of logistical difficulty. You must be prepared for it and build in time for issues that will force you to adjust your schedule. Remember, just because it is written on paper does not mean you must do the exact prescribed workout. You must allow flexibility, especially during this phase, because stressing over a missed workout could cause you to doubt all of the hard work achieved throughout the season. There is no reason to doubt your training because you miss one or two workouts. Always keep a very positive mental outlook.

Therefore, this portion of the schedule is the one you may not follow as closely. You should adapt it to your own individual situation, but you must do your best to maintain the TEAMS philosophy. Trevor and Rachel's schedules weren't perfect, but they followed this system of training the best they could, and they believed in what they were doing and the result was the best American junior time for 10km and the 2nd best Canadian women's 20km time.

Here is an example of the last few weeks for an elite high school athlete in the Peak Season phase:

Week	Monday	Tuesday	Wednesday	Thursday	Friday	Saturday	Sunday	Mileage
39	6km easy run	12km walk Zone #1	12km walk Zone #1	3km w-up Norwegian Fartlek 2km c-d / 6km easy run	OFF Flying	OFF Flying / 30 min easy run	12km walk Zone #1	69km Total
40	10km walk Zone #1	Speedwork 3km w-up 8 x 500m 90 seconds rest 2km c-d Zone #3	8km walk Zone #1	8km walk Zone #1	6km walk Zone #1	10,000m RACE	6km easy run	64km Total
41	OFF	8km walk Zone #1	12km walk Zone #1	15km walk Zone #1 / 6km easy run	12km walk Zone #1	3km w-up Norwegian Fartlek 2km c-d Zone #3 / 6km easy run	15km walk Zone #1	89km Total
42	12km walk Zone #1	Speedwork 3km w-up 5 x 2km 2 min rest 2km c-d Zone #3 / 5km easy run	15km walk Zone #1	12km walk Zone #1	12km walk Zone #1	3km w-up Norwegian Fartlek 2km c-d Zone #3	12km walk Zone #1	98km Total
43	12km walk Zone #1	8km walk with 8 x 1 min pickups	10km walk Zone #1	8km walk Zone #1	6km walk Zone #1	10,000m RACE	6km easy run	65km Total

You might be confused by the variation from week to week. Given the short peak season, you are accomplishing different goals with your training each week. Week #39 is your last hard week of training, fine tuning your engine to perform at its peak. Week #40 is a taper week that includes a race. Week #41 is a recovery week from your race. Week #42 is a solid training week and thus the mileage is much higher than the previous two weeks. Week #43 is again a taper and race week.

Advice for Choosing a College

Selecting the place where you are going to be spending the next four years of your life is not an easy task. The college decision is multifaceted; all aspects of your life will play a role in shaping your decision. There are five major things to consider:

- Academic goals
- Athletic goals

- Family proximity
- Financial situation
- Personality

As it has been more years since I have been in college than I care to admit, and Jeff Salvage has a biased perspective of being a college professor, we've asked current student and Olympic hopeful Maria Michta to give her perspective on selecting a college. She provided the following questions and answers to help define your specific collegiate needs.

What are your long-term academic goals?

The answer to this question is actually given best by answering the following three questions:

- What are your career interests?
- What major(s) will prepare for your desired career?
- What level of schooling will you need to enter the job market?

One of the main purposes of going to college is to earn a degree. However, the degree itself will not get you a job. No matter how prestigious the undergraduate school you go to your actual degree is worth no more than a piece a paper. Instead, what is most valuable is the knowledge you acquired and experiences you've gained that allowed you to earn your degree. This is what has prepared you, and hopefully qualified you, for the rest of your life and in your chosen career. While one shouldn't discount that a more prestigious school has many benefits and unique experiences, ultimately, what you put into college is what you get out of it. Choose an institution that provides you the most opportunities in your area of interest. Remember, while a small school with smaller classes offers more personal attention, it is at the expense of offering less diverse courses. Large universities can offer endless possible majors, numerous different facilities, but may treat you as just another Scantron lost among a sea of faces in an overcrowded auditorium.

If you don't know your ultimate career goals, don't worry. Many college freshman are equally confused. You can choose to be undecided or take a guess and choose a major which sounds interesting and then see how you like the required courses. Most college students have a general set of courses that are required regardless of your major. By taking the common courses and samples of some other courses of interest, you will be able to decide what major is right for you. As an undecided student athlete the more options you have the better. It may be wise to choose a setting that offers many different majors so you can keep your options open.

What are your long term athletic goals?

Student athletes have an additional set of criteria when evaluating potential schools. Once again it is important to think about what your goals are and what you require athletically to achieve your them.

What environment do you need to create athletically to achieve your goals?

Things to consider:

- School support system
- Coach
- Team
- Facilities
- Physical environment
- Weather
- Nearby terrain (i.e. a hilly mountainous campus is not conducive to race walking)
- Neighborhood Safety

As a race walker your first major question is: will I attend a college that has race walking in the conference program? The largest opportunity to compete for your college as a race walker is to attend an NAIA school. There are some NCAA schools which also offer race walk at the conference level but be aware there are no regionals or NCAA Nationals for race walkers. The benefit of selecting a school that competes at a conference level is you are automatically on the college team and will have opportunities to race directly for your school. This provides you with a team for support and a coach for guidance.

Be aware, however, not every school track coach knows enough about race walking to effectively coach an aspiring elite race walker. Therefore, you need to discuss with the coach at your college how he/she feels about you getting coaching from outside the university. This is easier than you think. Given today's technology, communicating with emails, cell phones, and cameras can help critique your form making your virtual coach seem like he/she is there. If your outside coach lives near your college this is even better.

Additionally, it is important to think about the benefit of having fellow teammates. Even if your teammates are not race walkers they can still be a great support system. Are you someone who needs structured practices at designated times with the support of teammates or can you wake up on cold mornings and workout alone? Knowing what you require to get out and train everyday is important in your decision making.

Another factor for consideration is the availability of training facilities. If you attend a college where you are on the athletic team this should not be an issue. However, many race walkers are not so lucky. Does your college have set times for general use of facilities i.e. track, pool, weight room? Does the college have an indoor track? This may not be so important if you go to school in the south, but anyone training in a New England winter knows the value of an indoor facility. This is why the climate and location of a school is also very important. How does the weather affect you? If you are coming from Maine and you go to school in Wisconsin it won't be a big deal for you, but if you are coming from Texas and travel to Maine you are going to be shocked. For myself, I spent half my college days injured. Part of the reason was all of those super cold days that we had to train outside or inside on the concrete basement floor of the school. If you are used to that weather, great! If you aren't, find someplace with weather more favorable to elite level training or at least has a high quality indoor track. When I was going to school, the nearest indoor facility we could train in was 35 miles away. If the weather was bad and we couldn't train outside, typically the weather was also too dangerous for us to be driving in the snow and wind to train indoors and then turn around and drive home. If your school has an indoor facility and there is bad weather, make sure you are able to utilize it.

When keeping in mind access to facilities, this includes the athletic trainers as well. As we have stressed throughout this book, consistency is the key to success. Aches and pains are bound to happen, especially for those athletes who are still developing. I have never known an athlete who was injury free throughout their entire career, so it is important you find a school which allows you access to some sort of medical facility so they can get you back on track as quickly as possible.

> Another important factor to consider is what are your family concerns and how far from home are you willing to live?

For some, living too far from home would be detrimental. I have seen numerous athletes who moved away from home to a dramatically different living environment who were incapable of adapting to their new surroundings. Only you can answer how close you need your family and familiar setting. Consider this carefully before selecting a school on the other side of the country.

> How will you finance your education?

For myself, I didn't want to strap my parents with the burden of paying off my education for the next 20 years, so I chose the school that was offering me an opportunity to race walk and an opportunity to have some of my education paid. Money can definitely feel like a limiting factor, but remember what you put into your college experience by how much you apply yourself, not how much you pay, will dictate how much you get out of it. Fortunately there are many different options to financing one's college education: parental contributions, academic scholarships, athletic scholarships, outside scholarships such as fellowships and grants.

> Are you able to withstand the rigors of having a 'new" life in college away from where you grew up and with a new coach and team around you?

No matter where you choose to go to college it's going to require a lot of mental strength, especially being a student athlete. How mentally tough are you? How much can you handle? The more up front you are with yourself now the better you will be able to answer these necessary questions to aid you in finding the right college to succeed both academically and athletically.

> What if I can't find a perfect school that fits all my needs?

Think about what is most important to you. What do you need to create the right environment for you to excel ? Can any of your priorities be adjusted?

For example, as a high school senior I wanted a school where I could study physical therapy with molecular biology as a fall back, train at an elite level as a race walker, be able to afford tuition without loans, and was prepared to train alone being coached by my trusted outside coach. By January of my senior year my parents informed me all the top schools I wanted to attend would cost too much money even with my scholarships. As you can imagine this was extremely frustrating, but I decided to choose a school that would allow me to compete for the college team while earning my degree and graduate debt free. While I was in the top 1% of my high school class and an Intel Science finalist, I could have chosen a number of high ranking schools. Instead, my college, C.W. Post, was only a tier three college. Nonetheless, I made the most of my academic experience and graduated valedictorian while simultaneously training at an elite level qualifying for the 2008 Olympic Trials. My hard work, extensive extracurricular activities and numerous academic accolades prepared me for acceptance into several graduate programs in biomedical sciences.

Where I received my bachelor degree from was not as important because I decided to pursue a career as a microbiologist, which required additional schooling. In this competitive job market the majority of college graduates require at least a master's degree. Therefore, I was able to use my undergrad time as a stepping stone both academically and athletically. Currently I am working on my new goals: earning my doctorate degree in Microbiology at Mount Sinai School of Medicine in NYC and training to qualify for the 2012 Olympics. My decision of which graduate school to attend once again required much thought and deliberation in order to once again maximize opportunity to achieve both my athletic and academic goals.

Process for Choosing a School

The process for selecting a school can be daunting, so follow these simple steps to help sort out your choices. Start by visiting the campus of universities that peak your interest. Nothing replaces visiting the school and seeing what it is like. You have to like it, because you are going to be living there for the next four years or more and it is going to shape the person you are for the rest of your life.

Talk to the coach. See firsthand whether or not their personality is compatible with yours. Do they come across as genuine and caring or do they make you feel like you are just one of many people on their team?

Talk to the other members of the track team. See what they say about the coach and the school, their opinion is likely the best barometer of the experience you will have if you attend the school.

More Resources

www.racewalk.com has a list of colleges and universities that support race walking. Check it out for the latest information.

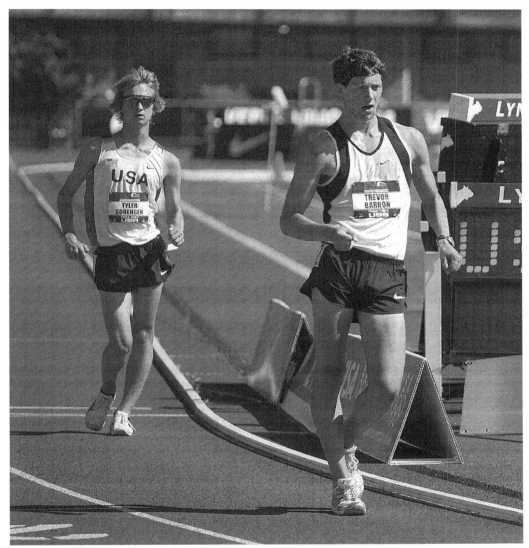

Trevor Barron Leading Tyler Sorensen at the 2009 10K U.S. Junior Nationals. The high school duo are both member of Champions International as well as two of America's biggest hopefuls.

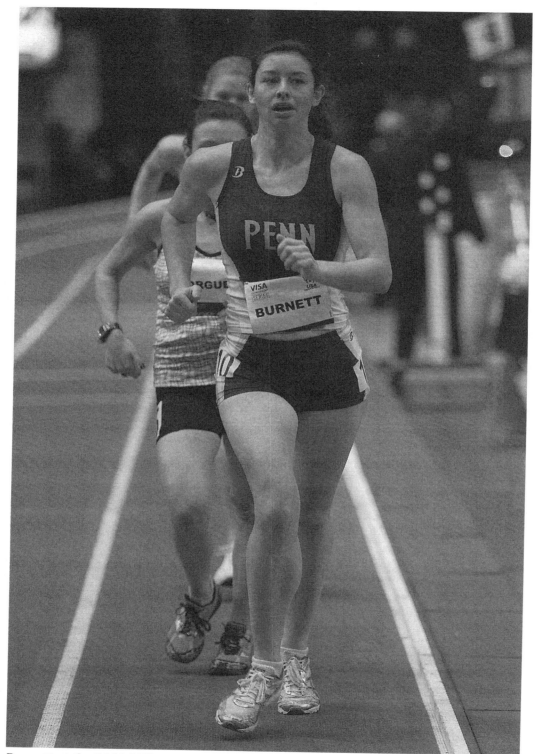

Katie Burnett at the 2010 Millrose Game is one of the leading Collegiate American Race Walkers

Chapter Six: Race Walking in College

When I graduated high school I was thankfully given an opportunity to receive a scholarship and attend the University of Wisconsin – Parkside in Kenosha, Wisconsin. At the time Parkside was in the National Association of Intercollegiate Athletics (NAIA) and I was given a tuition only scholarship – the most the school gave out. Some 15-plus years later schools are now offering full ride scholarships for athletes who can race walk and it is an opportunity that should not be overlooked. The race walk is a contested event at both the Indoor and Outdoor NAIA National Track and Field Championships and schools want to maximize the number of points that they can score. The race walk scores just as many points as any other event. Schools that want to win a national championship need points in every event that they can. Because of the current lack of depth, the race walk is an easy way to get them.

Receiving a scholarship for race walking was something that I didn't know existed until just a few months before my high school graduation. One of the reasons why we wanted to write this book was to give high school kids, their parents, and coaches the opportunity to know they too could have their college education paid for, but also to let them know that race walking in college is one way to propel them towards the Olympic Games. However, being on any athletic scholarship has both benefits and some difficulties.

The most important benefit is, of course, at the end of the four years you can graduate debt free. This helps if your ultimate goal is an Olympic Team berth as there are many other expenses incurred along that road. It also helps in life. If the Olympics aren't your ultimate path, you will enter the workforce without the burden of having to pay off your student loan for the next twenty years. Another benefit is the camaraderie you feel being part of a team atmosphere, which has always helped me reach my goals. It can help you as well. There were many days throughout my career where I just didn't want to go out and train. The weather was maybe too cold or there was some other "obstacle" to training, but having other people to train with got me out the door and on the road to improving. Training for longer distances is harder to do alone than the relatively short sprints in high school walking. Your team members will help make it easier. Finally, winning alone is nice, but when you win as part of a championship team the sweetness of victory will last forever.

While the benefits of a scholarship far outweigh the negatives, there are some issues to consider. For some young impressionable athletes, the pressure that they feel from their college coach to perform could be too much for them. College coaches, like all other coaches, want to succeed at their craft, and their craft is winning track and field meets. Some athletes crumble under this small amount of pressure; make sure you have an open line of communication with your coach, so they can put just the right amount of pressure to motivate you.

In addition, athletes training on a college team often must travel more frequently to school competitions. This usually results in missed classes as well as interrupting the training schedule. Often small college meets are required and the personal schedule is not considered when determining its value. Finally, for some schools, especially the smaller ones, there are inadequate medical support personnel with students being the "athletic trainers" in training. If your goal is to compete at an elite level, especially in an event like the race walk, knowledgeable athletic trainers and access to doctors is a must.

Overall, though, the thrill of being on scholarship and competing in college is priceless and worth any negatives that may occur. Race walking in college, particularly for those of you who go to an NAIA school, is a springboard for competing on the national level upon graduation. The NAIA Championships, both indoor and outdoor, are a great step along the way, but their distances are only 3,000m and 5,000m. Therefore, the long term focus of your training must be on the longer, more internationally recognized distances, particularly the 20km. Collegiate aged athletes are able to walk a great 5km race from 20km training, but flounder horribly if they train for the 5km and try and compete in the 20km. Chris Tegtmeier was the poster child for this type of training. Before he started training using the TEAMS philosophy, his sole focus was to walk fast in the 5km and try to win the NAIA Outdoor Championships. Chris's technique suffered greatly as he didn't have the endurance base required for a strong 20km effort. Chris would typically do shorter repeats and his longest training session of the season was just 12km. Chris had higher ambitions than just the NAIA National Championships, so Chris entered a few 20km races in the hopes of wearing red, white and blue at international competitions. While Chris was able to qualify for the team, every 20km for the rest of the season got progressively slower and even included a few trips to the medical tent. These near death experiences in Russia and Mexico made Chris realize that he needed to train differently. In 2009, Chris was able to walk a PR in the 5km at the NAIA Outdoor Nationals, while training for the 20km. More importantly, he was able to come back a few weeks later and walk a PR at the 20km Nationals to become the 7th fastest walker in America as well as establish himself firmly as the top collegiate male walker in the country. How did he do it? By increasing his endurance base and working the speed endurance component (Zone #2 and Zone #3) of his training, as opposed to pushing his body to exhaustion doing short repeats.

Race walking in college should be thought of as a progression. Each year builds upon the previous. For those of you who are utilizing the first collegiate schedule that follows, you should gradually increase your mileage after completing your first year under the TEAMS system. You should not feel that you have to go from this schedule to the elite schedule. It is about progression. That is the key to consistency of training and that is the key to *Race Walking Faster by Training Smarter*.

Developing a Schedule for Typical Collegiate Race Walkers

We present two training schedules for college athletes. One for a "typical" collegiate athlete who is looking toward the future in the 20km, but who currently needs to get strong enough at the 3km, 5km and 10km distances before progressing to longer distances. The second schedule is for the elite level collegiate athletes. These athletes have already proven themselves strong enough to handle the mileage necessary to compete well at the 20km, but who also want to succeed in the other distances as well, particularly in the 3km Indoor and 5km Outdoor NAIA National Championships.

As in the high school section, we have included some key holidays into the training program. With the TEAMS philosophy, it is very important all components of your life are taken into account. If a coach puts a certain type of workout onto the schedule, the athlete feels obligated to do the training that the coach prescribed. Therefore, it is very important to make sure you have either an easier workout or an off day during the holidays. This will ensure consistency of training and it will ensure a much more positive mental outlook for you in the weeks and months to come.

Phase I - Early Season Base Work for a Typical Collegiate Athlete:

The Early Season Base Work phase for a typical collegiate athlete lasts for seven weeks and starts around November 1st. These athletes usually progress from running cross country with their team and move over to walking toward the end of the fall season. The goal during this time is to increase your mileage while working on improving your technique. This will build a strong solid engine. To help fine tune it, focus on technique drills and stretching to increase your range of motion.

Here is a schedule for a typical collegiate level athlete:

Week	Monday	Tuesday	Wednesday	Thursday	Friday	Saturday	Sunday	Mileage
1	5km walk Zone #1	OFF	6km walk Zone #1	8km Hiking	OFF	8km walk Zone #1	10km Hiking	37km Total
2	8km walk Zone #1	6km run	10km walk Zone #1	10km Hiking	OFF	10km walk Zone #1	15km Hiking	59km Total
3	12km walk Zone #1	10km walk Zone #1	8km easy run	OFF	10km walk Zone #1 with 10 x 1 min pickups in the middle	12km walk Zone #1	15km Hiking	69km Total
4	8km walk Zone #1	2km w-up LACTATE TEST 6 x 2km 2km c-d	10km Hiking	12km walk Zone #1	OFF	15km walk Zone #1	15km Hiking	78km Total
5	10km walk Zone #1	12km walk Zone #1	15km walk Zone #1	OFF	10km progression walk – 1st 5km Zone #1, 2nd 5km Zone #2	18km walk Zone #1	20km Hiking	85km Total
6	10km walk Zone #1	12km walk Zone #1	15km walk Zone #1	OFF	10km run	18km walk Zone #1	20km Hiking	85km Total

Typically, a collegiate walker has finals the week before their holiday break. We have placed this as week # 7 in the schedule, but if your school is different adjust accordingly. Finals week is always a stressful time for students, but especially for student-athletes, as they have to balance the rigors of high academics and high athletics at the same time. Therefore, this is an especially important time not to over train. As recovery is the key to consistency of training, we decrease mileage by adding rest days so that you may take the time to study and rest. Listen to your heart rate during training and follow the paces prescribed. If you need to switch your days around, do so based upon your academic workload.

Week	Monday	Tuesday	Wednesday	Thursday	Friday	Saturday	Sunday	Mileage
7 Recovery Week Finals Week	OFF	12km walk Zone #1	OFF or 8km walk Zone #1	12km walk Zone # 1	OFF or 8km walk Zone #1 or easy run	Bohdan's Rhythm workout 6km easy run	18km walk Zone #1	76km Total

Phase II - Late Season Base Work for a Typical Collegiate Athlete

The Late Season Base Work phase lasts six weeks. The goal during this time is to increase your mileage while introducing slightly more intensity to prepare you for future harder workouts. This intensity is added in the form of longer fartleks and it is important not to increase the intensity of your Zone #1 workouts.

This phase culminates with the Millrose Games. Held on the last Friday in January for over 100 years, it was a staple competition for many throughout their career. If you are unable to qualify for this race, find another race to walk around that same weekend and adjust the schedule.

Week	Monday	Tuesday	Wednesday	Thursday	Friday	Saturday	Sunday	Mileage
8	10km easy run	12km walk Zone #1	15km walk Zone #1	Christmas Eve 8km easy run	Christmas Day OFF	Fartlek 3k w-up 8 x 500/500 2k c-d Zone #3 5km run	18km walk Zone #1	81km Total
9	8km easy run	Fartlek 3k w-up 3 x 2km/1km 2k c-d Zone # 3 4km easy run	16km walk Zone #1	10km walk Zone #1 New Years Eve	New Years Day OFF	8km walk Zone #1	3,000m Indoor qualifying race	66km Total
10	10km walk Zone #1	12km walk Zone #1 6km easy run	15km walk Zone #1	12km walk Zone #1 8km easy run	10km walk Zone #1	Fartlek 3k w-up 3 x 3km/1km 2k c-d Zone #2 6km easy run	15km walk Zone #1	101km Total

Week	Monday	Tuesday	Wednesday	Thursday	Friday	Saturday	Sunday	Mileage
11	8km walk Zone #1 or 8km easy run	10km Progression walk 1st - 5km Zone #1, 2nd - 5km Zone #2	10km walk Zone #1	12km walk Zone #1	Fartlek 3k w-up 2 x 3km/1km 2k c-d Zone #2/#3 6km easy run	18km walk Zone #1	10km walk Zone #1	87km Total
12	Mexican Speedwork 3km w-up 2 x 1000, 800, 600, 400, 200 2km c-d Zone 4 5km easy run	15km walk Zone #1	12km walk Zone #1	8km walk Zone #1 Or 8km easy run	Bohdan's Rhythm workout 3km w-up 4 x 100, 200, 300, 400 w/ 100m easy between 2km c-d Zone # 4 6km easy run	15km walk Zone #1	12km walk Zone #1	95km Total
13	Speedwork 3km w-up 10 x 500m 90 seconds rest 2km c-d Zone #3	12km walk Zone #1	12km walk Zone #1	8km walk Zone #1	3km AM pedestrain walk to loosen up 1-MILE Race Millrose Games	12km walk Zone #1	15km walk Zone #1	77km Total

Phase III - In Season Racing for a Typical Collegiate Athlete:

After week 13, the In Season Racing phase begins and the fun starts. After 13 weeks of working on your endurance, you are ready to work on the speed-endurance component of your training. There is a mixture of both longer and shorter fartleks to adapt your body to higher intensity walking. The longer fartleks get you stronger for extended periods of time, while the shorter fartleks improve your turnover. Since you probably will race at the NAIA Indoor Nationals, a few of the "Mexican Speedwork" sessions are included to tune your engine for a shorter speedy race.

Remember, the NAIA Indoor Nationals is not the peak of the season, it will just be one stop on the way to qualifying for and competing in the USATF Outdoor Track & Field Nationals and then, hopefully, the U.S. Olympic Trials.

During this phase, you will see some traditional races on the calendar. The NAIA Indoor and Outdoor Championships, the Penn Relays, as well as the approximate weekend for the World Cup or America's Cup Trials race. None of these races are over 20km. The World Cup or America's Cup is a 20km, but they have traditionally had an accompanying 10km race and that is what most of you should be shooting for at this point in the season. For this group, depending on your ability, you should probably stick with working on walking as fast as possible for 10km and under, and only walking a 20km at the USATF Outdoor Nationals if you are able to qualify at one of the alternative

91

distances such as 5km or 10km. The standards for men are 23:20 at 5km and 48:20 at 10km, while the women's standards are 26:00 for 5km and 54:00 for 10km. If you are not prepared to race a 20km in the middle of your season, the excessive stress can have a deadly effect on the rest of your season. There is plenty of time for longer races, once you've built up to them. Be patient and focus on the goals at hand.

If you have other races to compete in that are not included in this schedule, follow the taper and recovery weeks in chapter 3, but don't forget that all races need not have a full taper. Some races in college are entered solely to score points and they may become harder workouts instead of all out efforts. If you add a race as a workout, use it in place of one of the fartleks for the week.

You will notice the typical collegiate athlete isn't scheduled to compete in the USATF Indoor Championships a week before the NAIA Indoor Nationals. This is because typically for these athletes, it is better to focus on just one of the events. Trying to focus on both could mean lower overall results in both. So instead, focus solely on the NAIA Indoor Nationals, as you can only compete there four times.

Here is the In Season Racing phase for the typical collegiate athlete:

Week	Monday	Tuesday	Wednesday	Thursday	Friday	Saturday	Sunday	Mileage
14	OFF	Fartlek 3km w-up 8 x 500/500 2km c-d Zone #3 --- 6km easy run	15km walk Zone #1	12km walk Zone #1	6km run	Bohdan's Rhythm workout 3km w-up 4 x 100, 200, 300, 400 with 100m easy walking between 2km c-d Zone #3 / #4 --- 6km easy run	18km walk Zone #1	87km Total
15	8km walk Zone #1	2km w-up LACTATE TEST 6 x 2km 2km c-d --- 6km easy run	15km walk Zone #1	OFF	10km walk Zone #1	Fartlek 2km w-up 8 x 1km/500m 2km c-d Zone #3 --- 6km easy run	18km walk Zone #1	95km Total
16	8km walk Zone #1	Speedwork 3km w-up 3 x 3km 2:30 rest 2km c-d Zone #2/#3 --- 4km easy run	12km walk Zone #1	10km walk Zone #1	8km easy run	Mexican Speedwork 3km w-up 3 x 1000, 800, 600, 400, 200 2km c-d 2 min rest Zone #4 --- 6km easy run	16km walk Zone #1	92km Total

Week	Monday	Tuesday	Wednesday	Thursday	Friday	Saturday	Sunday	Mileage
17	8km walk Zone #1	Speedwork 3km w-up 4 x 2km 2:30 rest 2km c-d Zone #3 6km easy run	15km walk Zone #1	12km walk Zone #1	6km easy run	Mexican Speedwork 3km w-up 3 x 1000, 800, 600, 400, 200 2km c-d 2 min rest Zone #4 6km easy run	20km walk Zone #1	100km Total
18	10km walk Zone #1	Speedwork 3km w-up 4 x 2km 2:30 rest 2km c-d Zone #3 5km easy run	15km walk Zone #1	12km walk Zone #1	12km walk Zone #1	Speedwork 3km w-up 8 x 1km 2 min rest Zone #3 5km easy run	18km walk Zone #1	100km Total
19	12km walk Zone #1	Mexican Speedwork 3km w-up 2 x 1000, 800, 600, 400, 200 2km c-d 2 min rest Zone #4	12km walk Zone #1	8km walk Zone #1	6km walk Zone #1	Speedwork 3km w-up 5 x 1km 4 x 500m 2 min rest 2km c-d Zone #3 5km easy run	12km walk Zone #1	78km Total
20	OFF	Speedwork 3km w-up 8 x 500m 2 min rest 2km c-d Zone #3	10km walk Zone #1	8km walk Zone #1	5km walk Zone #1	NAIA Indoor Nationals	6km easy run	46km Total
21 Rec. Week	OFF	12km walk Zone #1	12km walk Zone #1	10km walk Zone #1	8km walk Zone #1	Fartlek 3km w-up 10 x 500/500 2km c-d Zone #3 5km easy run	18km walk Zone #1	80km Total
22	6km easy run	Speedwork 3km w-up 5 x 2km 2 min rest 2km c-d Zone #3	12km walk Zone #1	10km walk Zone #1	8km walk Zone #1	Speedwork 3km w-up 10 x 1km 2 min rest 2km c-d Zone #3 5km easy run	12km walk Zone #1	83km Total
23	12km walk Zone #1	Speedwork 3km w-up 8 x 500m 2km c-d Zone #3 5km easy run	10km walk Zone #1	8km walk Zone #1 Fly to race	6km walk Zone #1	10km RACE (World Cup Trials or America's Cup Trials)	8km easy run	73km Total

Week	Monday	Tuesday	Wednesday	Thursday	Friday	Saturday	Sunday	Mileage
24	OFF	12km walk Zone #1	12km walk Zone #1	8km easy run	10km walk Zone #1	Fartlek 3km w-up 10 x 500/500 2km c-d Zone #3	20km walk Zone #1	77km Total
25	10km walk Zone #1	Fartlek 3km w-up 4 x 2km/1km 2km c-d Zone #3 / 4km easy run	18km walk Zone #1	OFF	10km walk Zone #1	Speedwork 3km w-up 4km, 3km, 2km, 1km 3 min rest 2km c-d Zone #3 / 6km easy run	20km walk Zone #1	100km Total
26	10km walk Zone #1	Speedwork 3km w-up 6 x 1600m 2 min rest 2km c-d Zone #3	15km walk Zone #1	12km walk Zone #1	10km walk Zone #1	Speedwork 3km w-up 8 x 1km 2 min rest 2km c-d Zone #3	15km walk Zone #1	90km Total

Phase IV - Peak Season for a Typical Collegiate Athlete

The Peak Season phase for a typical collegiate athlete focuses on the NAIA Outdoor Championships. This is the time period where all of your hard work comes together and you perform at your best. Make sure you are getting enough sleep and eating properly. If the weather is hot, make sure that you abide by the concepts presented in chapter 11 for acclimatization, and drinking enough electrolytes.

Here is the Peak Season phase for a typical Collegiate Athlete:

Week	Monday	Tuesday	Wednesday	Thursday	Friday	Saturday	Sunday	Mileage
27	8km walk Zone #1	Speedwork 3km w-up 10 x 500m 90 sec rest 2km c-d Zone #3	10km walk Zone #1	OFF Or 6km walk Zone #1	6km walk Zone #1	PENN RELAYS 10km men 5km women	8km easy run	63km Total
28	OFF	10km walk Zone #1	12km walk Zone #1	10km walk Zone #1	10km walk Zone #1	Speedwork 3km w-up 8 x 1km 2 min rest 2km c-d Zone # 3	18km walk Zone #1	78km Total

Week	Monday	Tuesday	Wednesday	Thursday	Friday	Saturday	Sunday	Mileage
29	OFF	3km w-up Norwegian Fartlek 2km c-d Zone #3	15km walk Zone #1	12km walk Zone #1	12km walk Zone #1	Speedwork 3km w-up 3 x 2km, 4 x 1km 2:30 rest 2km c-d Zone #3	16km walk Zone #1	84km Total
30	8km walk Zone #1	Mexican Speedwork 3km w-up 3 x 1000, 800, 600, 400, 200 2 min rest 2km c-d Zone #4	15km walk Zone #1	10km walk Zone #1	Speedwork 3km w-up 8 x 1km 2 min rest 2km c-d Zone #3	12km walk Zone #1	10km walk Zone #1	82km Total
31	Speedwork 3km w-up 10 x 500m 90 seconds rest 2km c-d Zone # 3	8km walk Zone #1	8km walk Zone #1	6km walk Zone #1	NAIA Outdoor Nationals 5,000m	8km easy run	12km walk Zone #1	62km Total

Additional Phase for a Typical Collegiate Athlete:

We have also included a sample four week schedule after the NAIA Nationals for those of you who have met the alternative distance qualifying time and would like to try the 20km at the USATF Outdoor Nationals. While it may not be ideal to participate in your first 20km race at the National Championships, the way the system is set up now, it would be a great opportunity for you to get some exposure and experience in the longer distances.

Week	Monday	Tuesday	Wednesday	Thursday	Friday	Saturday	Sunday	Mileage
32	OFF	12km walk Zone #1	15km walk Zone #1	OFF	10km walk Zone #1	Fartlek 3km w-up 10 x 500/500 2km c-d Zone # 3	20km walk Zone #1	72km Total
33	12km walk Zone #1	Speedwork 3km w-up 6 x 2km 2:30 rest 2km c-d Zone #3 4km easy run	15km walk Zone #1	OFF	12km walk Zone #1	Speedwork 3km w-up 10 x 1km 2 min rest 2km c-d Zone #3 4km easy run	18km walk Zone #1	97km Total

Week	Monday	Tuesday	Wednesday	Thursday	Friday	Saturday	Sunday	Mileage
34	12km walk Zone #1	3km w-up Norwegian Fartlek 2km c-d Zone # 3	12km walk Zone #1	OFF	8km walk Zone #1	Speedwork 3km w-up 10 x 1km 2 min rest 2km c-d Zone # 3	10km walk Zone #1	73km Total
35	10km walk Zone #1	Speedwork 3km w-up 8 x 500m 2 min rest 2km c-d Zone #3	8km walk Zone #1	8km walk Zone #1	6km walk Zone #1	USATF Outdoor Nationals 20km RACE	8km easy run	59km Total

Developing a Schedule for Elite Collegiate Race Walkers

This schedule is the foundation for future training schedules of an Olympic level athlete. As a collegiate athlete you have a fairly flexible schedule with plenty of time throughout the day to squeeze in a few hours to get one, or two training sessions in a day. You just have to prioritize your schedule. I have seen many collegiate athletes over the course of my career tell me they didn't have time to train, but they did have time to go and "party" a few times a week. Sacrifices are necessary, but life is about choices. If you are an elite athlete in college you must make the sacrifices necessary to achieve your goals.

Phase I - Early Season Base Work for Elite Collegiate Athletes:

The Early Season Base Work phase for the elite collegiate athlete begins around October 1st. It lasts nine weeks and the goal is to get the athlete strong enough to handle the rest of the season. We chose this date because typically as an elite collegiate athlete you are on some sort of combined cross country and track scholarship and are required to compete in a few early season cross country races. Soon after the season starts, it would be wise for you to slowly transition to full-time walking. Throughout the phase there is a gradual build up in mileage. Most of this mileage is walked at Zone #1. You must have patience during this phase to make sure you do not walk too fast. Those who walk too fast during this phase are sure to peak too early. In addition, you will see some longer hikes on the schedule. These get your legs stronger and prepared for what is ahead.

Here is the Early Season Base Work phase for elite collegiate athletes:

Week	Monday	Tuesday	Wednesday	Thursday	Friday	Saturday	Sunday	Mileage
1	5km walk Zone #1	6km easy run	6km walk Zone #1	8km easy run	OFF	6km walk Zone #1	8km Hiking	39km Total
2	10km walk Zone #1	8km easy run	8km walk Zone #1	10km walk Zone #1	OFF	10km walk Zone #1	10km Hiking	56km Total
3	10km walk Zone #1	10km easy run	12km walk Zone #1	8km walk Zone #1	OFF	12km walk Zone #1	12km Hiking	64km total
4	8km walk Zone #1 / 6km easy run	10km easy run	12km walk Zone #1	10km walk Zone #1 / 5km easy run	OFF	15km walk Zone #1	15km Hiking	81km Total

Week	Monday	Tuesday	Wednesday	Thursday	Friday	Saturday	Sunday	Mileage
5	8km walk Zone #1 / 6km easy run	10km easy run	12km walk Zone #1	10km walk Zone #1 / 6km easy run	OFF	18km walk Zone #1	18km Hiking	88km Total
6	8km walk Zone #1	2km w-up LACTATE TEST 6 x 2km 2km c-d	16km walk Zone #1	12km walk Zone #1	10km easy run	20km walk Zone #1	18km Hiking	100km Total
7	12km walk Zone #1	10km Progression walk 1st - 5km Zone #1, 2nd - 5km Zone #2 / 6km easy run	15km walk Zone #1	12km walk Zone #1	10km easy run	20km walk Zone #1	15km Hiking	100km Total
8	10km walk Zone #1 / 6km easy run	10km walk Zone #1	15km walk Zone #1	12km walk Zone #1	8km walk Zone #1	12km Progression Walk 1st - 6km Zone #1, 2nd - 6km Zone #2 / 5km easy run	22km walk Zone #1	100km Total
9 Rec. Week	12km walk Zone #1 / 6km easy run	10km walk Zone #1	15km walk Zone #1	8km walk Zone #1	OFF	10km easy run	15km walk Zone #1	76km Total

Phase II - Late Season Base Work for Elite Collegiate Athletes

The Late Season Base Work phase lasts five weeks. The goal during this time is to increase your mileage while introducing slightly more intensity to prepare you for future harder workouts. This intensity is added in the form of longer fartleks and it is important to note not to increase the intensity of your Zone #1 workouts.

Longer fartleks are introduced for the first time, and these are done in Zone #2. This is to build up your strength, without peaking your body. The Millrose Games is also placed into the schedule, since this should be a staple for all elite collegiate athletes. Typically there is just one harder session per week during this phase, but we have thrown a few shorter fartleks into the schedule to keep things fresh and wake up your legs.

Here is the Late Season Base Work phase for elite collegiate athletes:

Week	Monday	Tuesday	Wednesday	Thursday	Friday	Saturday	Sunday	Mileage
10	12km walk Zone #1	12km walk Zone #1 / 6km easy run	15km walk Zone #1	12km walk Zone #1	8km walk Zone #1	Fartlek 3km w-up 3 x 4km/1km Zone #2 2km c-d / 6km easy run	20km walk Zone #1	106km Total
11	12km walk Zone #1	12km walk Zone #1 / 6km easy run	10km walk Zone #1	8km easy run	10km walk Zone #1	Fartlek 3km w-up 2 x 5km /1km Zone #2 2km c-d / 6km easy run	20km walk Zone #1	100km Total
12	18km walk Zone #1	12km walk Zone #1 / 6km easy run	15km walk Zone #1	Christmas Eve 8km easy run	Christmas Day Off	Fartlek 3km w-up 3 x 3km/1km Zone #2 2km c-d / 6km easy run	20km walk Zone #1	102km Total
13	12km walk Zone #1	Speedwork 2km w-up 12 x 500m 2 min rest 2km c-d	10km walk Zone #1	New Years Eve 10km walk Zone #1	New Years Day 8km easy run	6km walk Zone #1	3,000m INDOOR Qualifying race	62km Total
14	6km walk Zone #1	12km walk Zone #1	18km walk Zone #1	OFF	10km walk Zone #1	Fartlek 3km w-up 3 x 4km /1km Zone #2 2km c-d	20km walk Zone #1	86km Total

Phase III - In Season Racing for Elite Collegiate Athletes:

This phase spans from week #15 through just before the NAIA Outdoor Nationals. We have included a few staple races for you to compete in, but you will probably be required by your team to compete in a few more. This is not a big issue. You can adjust the schedule by following the taper week outlined in chapter 3. Remember though, not all races require a taper. The goal during this phase is to build up the speed endurance component of your training, while still competing in some less significant competitions.

The USATF Indoor Nationals and the NAIA Indoor Nationals are both on the schedule, but these do not have to be peaked for. You will be strong enough to compete in both races successfully because of the work you have completed over the previous few months.

Here is the In Season Racing phase for elite collegiate athletes:

Week	Monday	Tuesday	Wednesday	Thursday	Friday	Saturday	Sunday	Mileage
15	12km walk Zone #1	Mexican Speedwork 3km w-up 3 x 1000, 800, 600, 400, 200 2km c-d Zone #4 ⸺ 6km easy run	18km walk Zone #1	12km walk Zone #1	12km walk Zone #1	Fartlek 3km w-up 2 x 6km/1km Zone #2 2km c-d	20km walk Zone #1	113km Total
16	12km walk Zone #1	Mexican Speedwork 3km w-up 3 x 1000, 800, 600, 400, 200 2km c-d Zone #4 ⸺ 5km easy run	15km walk Zone #1	12km walk Zone #1	Bohdan's Rhythm workout 3km w-up 4 x 100, 200, 300, 400 w/ 100m easy between 2km c-d Zone #4 ⸺ 6km easy run	18km walk Zone #1	12km walk Zone #1	105km Total
17	Speedwork 3km w-up 10 x 500m 90 second rest 2km c-d Zone #3/#4 ⸺ 5km easy run	15km walk Zone #1	10km walk Zone #1	8km walk Zone #1	3km AM Pedestrian Walk ⸺ Millrose Games 1-Mile RACE	12km walk Zone #1	20km walk Zone #1	88km Total
18	OFF	Fartlek 3km w-up 10 x 500/500 2km c-d Zone # 3 ⸺ 6km easy run	12km walk Zone #1	12km walk Zone #1	12km walk Zone #1	3km w-up Norwegian Fartlek 2km c-d Zone # 3 ⸺ 6km easy run	22km walk Zone #1	100km Total
19	8km walk Zone #1	2km w-up LACTATE TEST 6 x 2km 2km c-d ⸺ 6km easy run	15km walk Zone #1	12km walk Zone #1	10km walk Zone #1	Fartlek 2km w-up 10 x 1km/500m 2km c-d Zone #3 ⸺ 6km easy run	25km walk Zone #1	106km Total

Week	Monday	Tuesday	Wednesday	Thursday	Friday	Saturday	Sunday	Mileage
20	8km walk Zone #1	Speedwork 3km w-up 3 x 4km 2:30 rest 2km c-d Zone #2/3 / 4km easy run	16km walk Zone #1	12km walk Zone #1 / 6km easy run	10km walk Zone #1	Fartlek 3km w-up 8 x 1km/500m 2km c-d Zone #3 / 6km easy run	25km walk Zone #1	121km Total
21	8km walk Zone #1	Speedwork 3km w-up 5 x 2km 2:00 rest 2km c-d Zone #3 / 6km easy run	18km walk Zone #1	12km walk Zone #1 / 6km easy run	12km walk Zone #1	Mexican Speedwork 3km w-up 3 x 1000, 800, 600, 400, 200 2km c-d 2 min rest Zone #4 / 6km easy run	25km walk Zone #1	122km Total
22	10km walk Zone #1	Fartlek 3km w-up 12 x 500/500 2km c-d Zone #3 / 5km easy run	15km walk Zone #1	12km walk Zone #1	12km walk Zone #1	Speedwork 3km w-up 10 x 1km 2 min rest Zone # 3	15km walk Zone #1	86km Total
23	12km walk Zone #1	Speedwork 3km w-up 12 x 500m 90 sec rest 2km c-d Zone #3	12km walk Zone #1	8km walk Zone #1	6km walk Zone #1	USATF Indoor Nationals 5,000m for men 3,000m for women RACE	16km walk Zone #1	75km Total
24	8km easy run	Speedwork 3km w-up 5 x 500m 2km c-d Zone #3	10km walk Zone #1	8km walk Zone #1	6km walk Zone #1	NAIA Indoor Nationals 3,000m RACE	8km run	56km Total
25 Rec. Week	OFF	8km walk Zone #1	12km walk Zone #1	10km easy run	6km walk Zone #1	3km w-up Norwegian Fartlek 2km c-d Zone #3 / 6km easy run	20km walk Zone #1	84km Total
26	8km easy run	Speedwork 3km w-up 6 x 2km 2 min rest 2km c-d Zone #3	15km walk Zone #1	12km walk Zone #1	10km walk Zone #1	Speedwork 3km w-up 6 x 1km 4 x 500m 2 min rest 2km c-d Zone #3 / 5km easy run	15km walk Zone #1	107km Total

Week	Monday	Tuesday	Wednesday	Thursday	Friday	Saturday	Sunday	Mileage
27	12km walk Zone #1	Speedwork 3km w-up 12 x 500m 90 seconds rest 2km c-d Zone #3 5km easy run	12km walk Zone #1	10km walk Zone #1	6km walk Zone #1	10km or 20km RACE (World Cup Trials or America's Cup Trials)	8km easy run	79km Total
28 Rec. Week	OFF	12km walk Zone #1	18km walk Zone #1	OFF	12km walk Zone #1	Fartlek 3km w-up 12 x 500/500 2km c-d Zone # 3	25km walk Zone #1	84km Total
29	12km walk Zone #1	Fartlek 3km w-up 5 x 2km/1km 2km c-d Zone #3 4km easy run	18km walk Zone #1	8km walk Zone #1	12km walk Zone #1	Fartlek 3km w-up 10 x 1km/500 2km c-d Zone #3 6km easy run	25km walk Zone #1	125km Total
30	8km walk Zone #1	Fartlek 3km w-up 5 x 2km/1km 2km c-d Zone #3 6km easy run	18km walk Zone #1	15km walk Zone #1	12km walk Zone #1	3km w-up Norwegian Fartlek 2km c-d Zone #3	22km walk Zone #1	116km Total
31	12km walk Zone #1	Speedwork 3km w-up 10 x 500m 90 sec rest 2km c-d Zone #3 5km easy run	18km walk Zone #1	OFF	10km walk Zone #1	PENN RELAYS 10km men 5km women	8km easy run	78km Total
32 Rec. Week	12km walk Zone #1	OFF	15km walk Zone #1	12km walk Zone #1	Fartlek 3km w-up 5 x 2km/1km 2km c-d Zone #3	22km walk Zone #1 5km easy run	12km walk Zone #1	97km Total
33	Speedwork 3km w-up 10 x 1km 2km c-d Zone #3 2 min rest	20km walk Zone #1	12km walk Zone #1	12km walk Zone #1	Fartlek 3km w-up 12 x 500/500 2km c-d Zone #3	18km walk Zone #1	12km walk Zone #1	106km Total

Week	Monday	Tuesday	Wednesday	Thursday	Friday	Saturday	Sunday	Mileage
34	Speedwork 3km w-up 3 x 2km 4 x 1km 2km c-d 2 min rest Zone #3	15km walk Zone #1	12km walk Zone #1	10km walk Zone #1	Mexican Speedwork 3km w-up 2 x 1000, 800, 600, 400, 200 with 2 min rest 2km c-d Zone #4	15km walk Zone #1	12km walk Zone #1	100km Total
	6km easy run				4km easy run			

Phase IV - Peak Season for Elite Collegiate Athletes:

The Peak Season phase for elite collegiate athletes is similar to the typical collegiate athlete. Both groups are going to be able to excel at 5km at the NAIA Outdoor National Championships. The difference is the elite collegiate athletes are going to also be prepared for the 20km a few weeks later at the USATF Outdoor Nationals.

The USATF Outdoor Nationals should be the ultimate goal for all collegiate athletes. The opportunity to compete with Olympic level athletes is an extraordinary experience for these athletes. The first time I competed in the USATF Outdoor Nationals, the meet was held in Eugene, Oregon, the home of Steve Prefontaine. The feeling of electricity was in the air. You, too, can have the same experience.

Here is the Peak Season phase for elite collegiate athletes:

Week	Monday	Tuesday	Wednesday	Thursday	Friday	Saturday	Sunday	Mileage
35	Speedwork 3km w-up 12 x 500 90 sec rest 2km c-d Zone #3	12km walk Zone #1	10km walk Zone #1	6km walk Zone #1	NAIA Outdoor Nationals 5,000m	8km easy run	15km walk Zone #1	72km Total
36 Rec. Week	OFF	12km walk Zone #1	15km walk Zone #1	Fartlek 3km w-up 12 x 500/500 2km c-d Zone # 3	22km walk Zone #1	12km walk Zone #1	15km walk Zone #1	93km Total
37	12km walk Zone #1	Speedwork 3km w-up 6 x 2km 2 min rest 2km c-d Zone # 3	15km walk Zone #1	12km walk Zone #1	12km walk Zone #1	Speedwork 3km w-up 12 x 1km 2 min rest 2km c-d Zone #3	20km walk Zone #1	113km Total
		4km easy run				4km easy run		

Week	Monday	Tuesday	Wednesday	Thursday	Friday	Saturday	Sunday	Mileage
38	12km walk Zone #1	3km w-up Norwegian Fartlek 2km c-d Zone #3 / 6km easy run	18km walk Zone #1	10km walk Zone #1	6km walk Zone #1	Speedwork 3km w-up 10 x 1km 2 min rest 2km c-d Zone #3 / 5km easy run	12km walk Zone #1	100km Total
39	12km walk Zone #1	Speedwork 3km w-up 10 x 500m 90 seconds rest 2km c-d Zone #3	10km walk Zone #1	8km walk Zone #1	6km walk Zone #1	USATF Outdoor Nationals 20km	8km easy run	79km Total

Non-NAIA Collegiate Athletes

Many race walkers chose to go to an National Collegiate Athletic Association (NCAA) university instead of an NAIA institution. There is nothing that says you can't go to an NCAA school and be successful. Many athletes have come up through these ranks and have had highly successful careers. The biggest issue is that the NCAA does not recognize race walking and therefore schools offering to help race walkers are subject to punitive fines. This was the case for one NCAA school which received a fine of $2,500 for helping one of their up-and-coming athletes travel to a national class competition.

While this may seem like a big detractor, it actually opens up a unique opportunity for those elite athletes who are good enough to win prize money. Since the NCAA does not recognize race walking, student-athletes who attend an NCAA university are able to accept prize money unlike their brethren on the track team. This does not even jeopardize their opportunity to compete in other sports, such as cross country.

Two great examples of athletes who attended NCAA schools and were able to excel were Maria Michta and Curt Clausen. Maria attended C.W. Post on Long Island, while Curt attended Duke University in North Carolina. Maria's coach was understanding and allowed her to run cross country in the fall and race walk for the rest of the year. For Clausen, he was allowed to wear a Duke jersey and had access to the facilities just like any other member of the track and field team. Maria is just beginning to make her mark on the national scene, while Clausen, after his days at Duke, went on to be America's only medal winner at the IAAF World Championships, earning a bronze medal in 1999.

If you choose to attend an NCAA institution, pick the school that is the best fit for your educational needs while close to a coach and at a training locale that is conducive for elite training. Zac Pollinger is a perfect example of an athlete not selecting a good environment for his athletic endeavors. Pollinger was one of the few U.S. Juniors in history to break 45:00 for 10km and had the talent to continue his race walking to the elite senior level, but his educational choice of going to

Harvard stopped his athletic aspirations in their tracks. Without a supportive group, Zac was unable to balance his education, social and athletic aspirations and moved away from his athletic dreams; thus America lost a potential future champion. When you decide on a college, chose one that will enable you to accomplish both your academic and athletic goals at the same time if you would like to continue to excel as a track and field athlete.

Tales from the Track – Lauren Forgues

I will never forget the time when I was competing in the Junior division of the Pan-American Race Walking Cup in Brazil. It was the end of my freshmen year at the University of Maine and I focused my training toward this race all season. The year before I failed to make the Junior World Cup team so I was very motivated to make the Junior Pan American team. Balancing school and training was a difficult feat, but I was very focused on my athletic and academic goals. In college it is very easy to become distracted by all of your new found freedoms, but I found a good balance between training, school and having a little fun. Because the University of Maine was an NCAA school, they were not allowed to fund my race walking aspirations. However, I ran cross country in the fall and the coach graciously continued to work with me for the track season. My coach did not have any clue how to coach a race walker, so with help from Dr. Tom Easter, Tim Seaman and other race walking gurus, I was able to train for the trials race. In March, my dad and I flew to Miami to compete in the trials race where I smoked the competition and walked my Junior PR of 50:30 for 10k.

In Brazil, I was star struck. It was the first time that I was on the same team with Olympian Kevin Eastler and I was so excited. The junior women's race was in the middle of the afternoon and the sun was very hot that day. I knew I wanted to walk fast, but I did not expect to perform as well as I did. The gun went off and the South Americans surged ahead. I did not go out as fast as the lead pack but I found myself in the middle, alone. As the kilometers ticked by, I found myself inching closer and closer to the lead pack. As the sun bore down, I started passing my South American competitors. With one lap left I continued to pick off the deteriorating lead pack. Tim Seaman and Kevin Eastler were screaming at me to keep going, as I was walking into medal position. With one kilometer to go I saw the third place girl swaying ahead, the heat was too much for her. With the finish line in sight, I laid the hammer down and passed her, cruising across the finish line slightly behind 2nd place and earning the bronze medal. I finished just a minute slower than my PR but more importantly, I earned the only medal for Team USA. That race set me up for many more successes and was a good taste of what competing at an international level is like. It taught me not to limit my goals.

Participating on a Varsity Cross Country Team

For those of you on your varsity cross country team, you should not feel you are sacrificing too much to be an elite collegiate level race walker. You are gaining a great cardiovascular base from your cross country program that pays dividends later. Be patient and do not rush your conversion back to full-time race walking by just jumping into the middle of the schedule or by cutting short your cross country season. You can adapt the Early Season Base Work phase and Late Season Base Work phase to your unique situation. The biggest mistake you can make is to go straight from cross country and start walking fast by skipping the early part of the training cycle. Start off slow because you do not want to risk an injury by calling on different muscles you haven't used in a while to start working harder than they are ready.

A great example of this was the senior year of Amber Antonia. Amber was not just one of the top runners at the University of Wisconsin – Parkside, she was the fastest runner ever for the school. She broke school records running that people thought wouldn't be broken for generations, and then she went on to become an equally successful race walker. She race walked her way to 1st place at the NAIA Outdoor Nationals and placed 3rd at the USATF 20km Outdoor Nationals when she was just 23 years of age. She ran faster than three-time Olympian Michelle Rohl. Amber was able to balance the rigors of high level cross country running and then go on and walk some impressive times for a collegiate athlete, times that could win most national championship races. Amber had to balance the requirements of her cross country scholarship with her desire to be an elite level race walker. If Amber was able to do it in her senior year, so can you.

Other Opportunities Beyond the National Championships

There are many other opportunities to compete after the national championships. Your season does not need to end with the return trip from the NAIA Outdoor Nationals or the USATF Outdoor Nationals. While our schedules do not continue past the Nationals, that should not be an excuse to go surfing every day. Instead, pick another goal and keep training. Fashion your post national schedule based upon your goal, but make sure to walk for a few weeks following the Late Season Base Work phase schedule with a few more weeks of the In Season Racing Phase as you approach your final races.

Here are a few of the races that you could try:

- The USATF Club Championships – Open to all athletes
- The World Junior Championships for those who are 19 years of age or under.
- The Pan-American Junior Championships, also for those who are 19 years of age or under.
- The North American, Central American, Caribbean Championships, typically called NACAC, for those athletes under 23 years of age.
- USATF 15km Championships. A nice transition to work your way up toward the longer distances.
- European races – go to www.european-athletics.org and see their schedule of races. While it may be far to travel, it would be a great opportunity for you to compete against other athletes. Try and get some local club members to sponsor your quest to go to Europe.
- Other domestic races – check out www.usatf.org and www.racewalking.org for a schedule of more races.

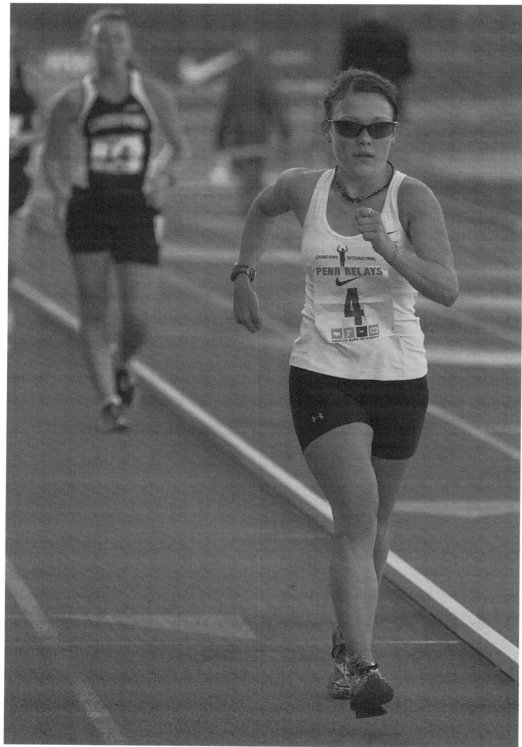

Lauren Forgues, of Champions International, at the 2010 Penn Relays. Soon after she walked a 1:40 20km, putting her within reach of the Olympic "B" standard.

Chapter Seven: Training for the Olympics

What it Takes

"If it were easy, everyone would make the Olympics," one-time U.S. Olympic hopeful Paul Schwartzberg once said. He was right. A great many factors must synergize for an elite athlete to evolve into an Olympian. Desire is first and foremost. Brooks Johnson, coach of many Olympic medalists, once told me that an athlete must have "five-ring fever" to be successful at the Olympic Games. Five-ring fever is the desire of an athlete to sacrifice everything to perform at his or her best for their country at the Olympic Games. Desire of course is not enough, or there would be many more Olympians. Mental fortitude and an innate ability not to get injured are also required. However, I feel Coach Enrique Peña summed it up best when he stated **"an Olympic Medal is not won, it is constructed."** It takes a team of people surrounding an Olympic hopeful to help him/her accomplish their dream of competing and performing well in the Olympic Games. It also takes talent, a supportive club, an understanding family, a team, a qualified coach and of course financial resources.

You've Got to Have Talent

Let's face the reality, not everyone is given the ability to win an Olympic Gold medal. If you are struggling to walk under ten-minute miles, you're probably not going to make the Olympic team. Sure, hard work, grit, and determination will get you far, but there are limits to what willpower can do. The same can be said for the limits of talent. Even the most talented person, without the right tools around him/her will not be able to become an Olympian. Many times I have seen extremely gifted athletes making mistake after mistake because they weren't doing things properly. Maybe they weren't stretching enough or maybe they weren't eating right. It doesn't matter what they were doing wrong, what they were doing wasn't allowing themselves to move forward toward being the best athlete they could be. Thus, they were inhibiting their chances to excel on the world stage. If you are going to be an Olympian, you can't waste your talent.

If I had to think of one athlete who didn't have a lot of natural talent, but was able to overcome this, it would be Andrew Hermann. Andrew himself would agree with this statement. Andrew didn't have the natural zip in his stride that those around him had. He didn't look very fluid when he race walked and he didn't have the speed necessary to walk the shorter distances. What Andrew did have was the ability to withstand the training necessary to be successful at the 50km. His ability to walk mile after mile without tiring was amazing and what led him to the status of Olympian.

A Supportive Family

The road to the Olympics is paved with many ups and downs. This is where a supportive family is extremely important. While the lone wolf can qualify without one, a nurturing family is a huge asset. Over the course of my career I could not have asked for a more understanding family. I remember my Dad's encouragement as we flew across the country to compete in my first Junior National Championships. Moments like these are priceless. Equally priceless were the tears of joy streaming down the cheeks of my mother and sister when I qualified for my first Olympic Team. Almost four years to the day earlier I saw them crying tears of sadness as I came across the finish line at the Olympic trials. Sadly, they realized that my second place finish meant that I had failed to qualify for the 1996 team. Having them there in 1996, 2000, and in 2004, allowed me to push my body to its maximum ability. Hearing them cheering so loudly as I walked around and around the course hoping to qualify for the Olympic team and represent our country, state, town and of course, our family on the world's biggest stage really helped. Equally important, they completely supported my sacrifice to pursue athletics instead of a traditional career. Many parents are not fond of their child giving up the financial rewards of a customary job for the glory of a non-revenue generating sport. Constant negativity is not the key to an Olympic berth. My parents excelled in the positive.

Today some of our young walkers are well supported by their parents. Tyler and Nicolette Sorensen's father Lars runs many of the workouts with them, as does Maria Michta's mom Sue. This support transcends borders as my wife Rachel's parents Nil and Christine have logged thousands of miles alongside her. Assistance like this is invaluable, especially if there isn't a team around with which to train.

A supportive family is like the roots of a tree; the stronger and bigger the roots, the less likely the tree will topple over when there are stormy times.

Being Part of a Team

Training by yourself is a lonely solitary affair. A sole walker finds it difficult to push his/her body to the levels necessary week after week. Teammates make it much easier to get out the door and put in the mileage necessary to qualify for the Olympic Games. It also makes it easier to walk the times necessary on the harder speed endurance sessions. The life of a solitary race walker can be quite boring, but being able to go out and meet your friends for a workout is going to help a lot. It is important to note there must be a positive environment amongst the members of the team. Many times in my career I have seen internal strife within the team tear it apart to the detriment of all parties. If you can't train every day with people, it is important to find someone to workout with you at least occasionally. This person can even be a runner or bicyclist. Ever since my high school graduation, whenever I am home on Long Island, my high school coach Frank Manhardt rode his bicycle with me thousands of miles around the streets of Brightwaters. Rain or shine, this now 82-year-old man rode next to me, talking to me about technique, training and about trying to make the Olympic Team. While Coach Manhardt can't ride his bike with all of you, find a positive supportive person to help you with your training.

Staying Healthy

Although many people gravitate to race walking because of the low incidence of injury, the reality is when you train 80 to 100 miles per week, injuries will occur. I have had three surgeries over my career with my last one taking me out of contention for the 2008 Olympic team. To train at an Olympic level your body therefore must be strong enough to withstand the training. Jeff Salvage had a lot of talent, but his body was not able to withstand the training necessary. In his short five-year elite race walking career he had three hernia operations, a car accident that injured his neck, and knee surgery. What magnified his issues were these injuries occurred when he was young and resilient. If you are going to make and excel at the Olympics, you must have a natural resistance to injury.

Having a Strong Mind

Another factor that influences an athlete performing well is his/her mental strength. One of the best examples of a U.S. athlete who epitomizes such fortitude is Curt Clausen. Curt was able to push his body to amazing levels of discomfort, while still being able to perform at a very high level. Elite race walkers may make it look easy, but walking at a world class level is always hard work. So many times in Curt's career he was able to overcome circumstances that would have crippled other human mortals, but not Clausen. In May 2000 Curt was competing in a 20km track event in Bergen, Norway, when he heard a popping sound. Curt was on American Record pace and he was determined to break the record which, yours truly, owned. The popping noise was Curt's meniscus tearing, but Curt was so determined to break my record he walked the last half of the race in pain every step of the way. Few people could have done that without tears running down their cheeks.

Never underestimate the human mind and the will power that it can unleash. If you don't believe you can do something, you will never achieve it. Have confidence in yourself and your training program. If you allow doubt to creep into your mind, you will wither under the pressure it takes to qualify for the Olympic Games.

Make sure the confidence you are required to have is an inward confidence. Don't tell people how great you are going to be, show them how great you are by achieving your goals. Outwardly confident people are construed as arrogant, and arrogance produces enemies. One of the most famous quotes ever was from the movie *The Godfather*. The Don stated, "Keep your friends close and your enemies closer." You will make enemies quickly with those around you if your confidence gets construed as arrogance.

Show Me the Money

Athletes in non-revenue generating events like race walking find it very difficult to fund their achievements. Without a major sponsorship, the bottom line is that it is the athlete, or their family, who bears the inevitable financial burden of trying to qualify for the Olympic Games. This does not mean you have to be rich to be an Olympian. Contrarily, the athlete must have access to and be willing to use some sort of "line of credit." If an athlete does not have an easy access to funds to pay for the items necessary to be an elite-level athlete, and if he/she does not have a federation which throws thousands of dollars their way, he/she will be unable to continue. The best example of this was when Will Van Axen was at the Olympic Training Center. Van Axen was one of the most talented American race walkers ever, but he lacked financial wherewithal to make it to the Games. At the end of the 1997 season, our training group was located at the Olympic Training Center in Chula Vista, California. Due to financial issues, we were trying to determine a way to keep Bohdan Bulakowski as our coach. The proposed solution was for each of the athletes to be responsible for coming up with $2,000 a year to subsidize Bohdan's salary. It seemed very reasonable for us and all but Van Axen agreed. Instead, Van Axen decided it was too much for him and he decided to "retire" at just 22 years of age. A few months later the North American Race Walking Institute (NARI) stepped in and took on the financial responsibility of paying for Bohdan's salary. They saved the group from certain destruction, but unfortunately Van Axen had already left the group. His inability to withstand the economic pressure was one of the reasons why America lost one of its greatest athletes before his time.

Another example of financial issues is a floating line of credit you may need. It was one of the most important sacrifices I had leading up to qualifying for my first Olympic team. I traveled to Cuenca, Ecuador, for a month for our altitude training camp; to Mexico to compete in a huge hemispheric championship, than a week later turned around and left for Europe for a seven-week, four-country tour. The vast majority of the financial burden was bore by my credit cards, and after I returned from representing my country on the world's biggest stage in front of 120,000 people, I had over $15,000 at 18% interest on my credit cards with only $1,000 in the bank. The "cost" of my first Olympic Team was tremendous, but it was something that was completely necessary and I would do over again if I had to because competing in the Olympics was an amazing experience. There would have been no way to make the Olympic team without this "access" to these funds.

A Club or Sponsor Makes the Difference!

One way to defer the personal cost is with a supportive club that can assist with airfare or other expenses associated with being an elite athlete. For me, the New York Athletic Club (NYAC) was the difference between making the Olympic Team and watching it on TV. Before Paul Mascali, the Track and Field Chairmen for the past 20 years, asked me to join the team, I had one American record and one national championship title. I now currently hold ten American records at varying distances and forty-three national championships. Without their help, the Olympic Games would have been just another unrealized dream for a middle class kid from the suburbs. Not only did the NYAC support me financially, they were also a sense of pride for me. Wearing NYAC across my chest enabled me to know there were thousands of club members who I represented in my quest to be an Olympian. When I finally qualified to be an Olympian, they were thrilled beyond belief and felt joy in my accomplishment. You, too, can feel the same by finding a club in your area that is supportive in achieving your dreams.

Is it Worth it?

The one question I am asked over and over again is, "was all of the sacrifice worth it?" The answer is whole heartedly, yes! The Olympics are the pinnacle of athletic competition. It's where the best of the best compete. There is no higher level of sports competition in the world. Billions of people watch and hope their athlete is able to rise to the level and perform at his or her best. In the Olympics anything can happen and almost anyone who qualifies has a chance at the gold.

The title of Olympian once given can never be taken away. As you march toward your dream of wearing the colors of your country across your chest, you have to remember you have a chance to make history. But with history, comes responsibility. Do you want to make history? That is a question that only you can answer.

My new year's resolution for 1995 was to do everything I could to make the 1996 Olympic Team. I had just a year and a half and the biggest challenge facing me would be to improve upon my 1:30:00 personal best time, a time I hadn't accomplished since 1993, to achieve the Olympic qualifying standard of under 1:26:00. This was a tall order, because my first race in March 1995 was nearly 1:40:00. I had literally started 1995 in horrendous walking shape. By June I had improved to 1:29:21 and placed 5th at the Outdoor Nationals -- just barely fast enough to qualify for the 1996 Olympic Trials, but still far away from a sub 1:26:00. I continued my normal training routine of three days of week doing one long walking session, one speedwork session and one tempo/long intervals/or race, with three days of running (normally eight miles aerobic/easy). I did this through December but felt I was not quite progressing fast enough. I called Mitch Craib, a physiologist at the Olympic Training Center in Colorado Springs, to discuss my training. His immediate response when I discussed my training was "Get rid of the running" and substitute race walking. His point was that in order to be the best I needed to be doing as much specific training as possible and because I had a tight work/training schedule, since I was working a full-time job, which did not allow me enough time to do both. I clearly was not training enough miles per week to be incorporating any running into my schedule. I had thought running made a lot of sense in that it gave my race walking muscles a bit of a break while still gaining cardiovascular benefits. Mitch disagreed. His advice was the best I could have gotten. The additional specific training I was able to do was likely the sole reason I was able to drop down to 1:25:40 by March and set myself up to win the Olympic Trials and make the U.S. Team. While I didn't have the race I wanted at the Olympic Games, I was inspired to continue to train and I knew the best was yet to come for myself as an athlete.

Curt Clausen is a three-time Olympian, World Championship Bronze Medalist and American 50km Record Holder.

What Does it Take to Make the Olympic Team?

In addition to all of the internal and external factors described previously, it takes thousands and thousands of miles of race walking to accomplish your dream of walking into the Olympic Stadium during the Opening Ceremonies. Consistency of training, having your days revolve around your training, and making sure you get enough recovery time, are the keys to successful training.

Coach DeWitt, my college coach from the University of Wisconsin – Parkside, used to tell us that almost every athlete who makes the Olympic Team didn't do it on his or her first time competing at the Olympic Trials. As a young athlete graduating college and as the first four-time NAIA Collegiate Champion, I did not want to hear this, but hindsight is 20/20 and Coach DeWitt was correct. In the last 30 years, no race walker who qualified for the Olympic Team did so in their first time competing at the Olympic Trials, with the sole exception of Yueling Chen, who eight years earlier was the first women's race walk Olympic Champion from China.

How Do You Qualify for the Olympics?

This is one of the most common questions asked and one of the most perplexing answers I have to give. When people ask me this question and they hear the answer, the look upon their faces is typically utter dumbfoundedness and confusion. Before 1992, if you finished in the top three positions at the Olympic Trials you qualified for the Olympic Team. It was that simple. Sadly this is no longer the case. Instead a myriad of rules and regulations must be read and studied. Even after reading them, many athletes cannot grasp what is being required of them. The IAAF (International Association of Athletic Federations) have two standards known as "A" and "B." The "A" standards for 20km are 1:22:30 for men and 1:33:30 for women, while the "B" standards are 1:24:20 for men and 1:38:00 for women. A country can send up to three athletes if all of the athletes have achieved a time faster than the "A" standard in a properly sanctioned race. If a country has one or more athletes with a "B" standard or just one "A" and one or more "B" standards, they are allowed to send just one athlete. If there is just one "A" standard athlete, even if that athlete is the World Record holder, and they get beat by the "B" standard athlete at the Olympic Trials – the "B" standard athlete gets to walk proudly into the Olympic stadium instead of his/her faster brethren.

While this is confusing, it is better than the alternative put forth by some countries for athletes to be sent to the Olympic Games. These athletes must be capable of placing in the top 8 or top 12 finishers. This is typically determined by a time standard, which is much faster than the "A" standard and a committee voting on whether or not to send the athlete or crush their dreams and aspirations.

Can you imagine walking a time faster than the "A" standard and faster than even the standard put forth by your country's Olympic Committee and then being told that you can't go? This system is utilized by the Canadians, Norwegians and many other European countries. In 1996, Kjersti Plaetzer was training for the Olympic Games in Atlanta. That year the times were super fast thanks to some great weather and good competition at a few races in Europe. Kjersti had walked a time of 44:40 in the 10km and historically raced very well in the heat. Unfortunately she was prohibited by her Norwegian Federation from competing because they thought that she wasn't fast enough. The race was still 10km with the eventual winner, Yelena Nikolayeva walking 41:49 to claim the gold. To put it in perspective, U.S.A.'s Michelle Rohl finished 14th in a time of 44:29. With a chance of being top 15, you are just not good enough for the Norwegian Olympic Team. While we will never know how Kjersti would have fared, we do know she would go on to walk 41:16 in 2003 and become the 2nd fastest 10km female walker in history. She also went on to win two Olympic silver medals, one in 2000 and another in 2008. When the pressure was on, Kjersti excelled. Under the U.S. system she would have qualified for her first Olympic Team in 1996 instead of 2000.

Developing a Schedule for Olympic Hopefuls

The following is a sample training schedule for a 20km athlete hoping to make the Olympic Team. The schedule is based not only on what I did as I made my way toward the 2004 Olympic Team, but also what I have learned along the way.

This schedule includes a double peak. It is the first schedule in the book to include two peaks in the same season. Peaking twice in the same season is a tough thing for a coach and an athlete to accomplish, but it is a necessity if you are going to compete in the Olympics. The first peak is going to be for the middle to the end of May. Typically this will be for an international race in Europe or the IAAF World Cup. Since the Olympic "A" and "B" standards are tough to obtain, the first peak will be for you to obtain the standard and the second peak will be for the Olympic Trials and the Olympic Games.

When we made up this schedule, we focused it on athletes hoping to obtain the IAAF "B" Standard. Since we have few people in the U.S. who have walked these standards, one of the obvious goals in writing this book was for us to help those athletes who are close to achieving their dream and actually achieve it. The schedule can easily be adapted for those athletes who are already at the "B" standard to obtain the "A" standard. Depending on the athlete, you can add some longer walks into the schedule, but the biggest thing is to just follow the TEAMS philosophy and walk in the zones prescribed.

Phase I - Early Season Base Work for an Olympic Level Athlete:

The Early Season Base Work phase for an Olympic level athlete is very critical. With a double peak for the season, it is important to get a solid base so you can build your engine for the entire season. During this phase, the goal for these athletes is going to be to get stronger and more flexible. The season is very long, so nothing fast is done during this phase. Weight and core training should be accomplished two to three times a week. There will also be a gradual build up in the distance by including both Zone #1 walks and hikes. When you are hiking, try to find some place which is challenging so you can naturally build up the strength in your legs. As three-time Olympian and American Record holder Curt Clausen has told me many times, hiking is about time on your feet. Allowing your body to adapt to moving for two to three hours is going to pay huge dividends later in the season. Also, when you are walking, try and find courses to walk on that aren't perfectly flat. I will never forget the first time I was in Flagstaff training with Team Plaetzer. Coach Stephan Plaetzer was driving a car next to us and he asked me how my heart rate was. I told him that it was a bit higher than I would expect because of the hilly course we are training on. He said, "Hills? What hills? These are bumps!" A few months later I went to Norway and saw the roads they train on and indeed, Flagstaff was "flat" compared to the town of Softeland where they train. Training on a hilly course, especially during the Early Season Base Work phase, is a great investment for later in the season. I have included an altitude training camp for four weeks during this phase. If you are seriously training to qualify for the Olympics, do not skip this. It will really help you to build up your engine and prepare it for the months ahead.

Here is the Early Season Base Work phase for an Olympic level athlete:

Week	Monday	Tuesday	Wednesday	Thursday	Friday	Saturday	Sunday	Mileage
1	6km walk Zone #1	8km easy run	8km walk Zone #1	OFF	8km walk Zone #1	10km walk Zone #1	10km Hiking	50km Total
2	8km walk Zone #1	12km easy run	10km walk Zone #1	OFF	10km walk Zone #1	12km walk Zone #1	15km Hiking	67km Total

Week	Monday	Tuesday	Wednesday	Thursday	Friday	Saturday	Sunday	Mileage
3	10km walk Zone #1	12km easy run	12km walk Zone #1 / 5km easy run	OFF	12km walk Zone #1	15km walk Zone #1	18km Hiking / 6km easy run	90km Total
4	12km walk Zone #1	12km walk Zone #1 / 6km easy run	15km walk Zone #1	OFF	12km walk Zone #1 / 5km easy run	18km walk Zone #1	20km Hiking / 5km easy run	108km Total
5	12km walk Zone #1	2km w-up LACTATE TEST 7 x 2km 2km c-d / 6km easy run	15km walk Zone #1	12km walk Zone #1 / 6km easy run	8km walk Zone #1 / 8km easy run	20km walk Zone #1	20km Hiking	125km Total
6	TRAVEL TO ALTITUDE / 8km Hiking	12km walk Zone #1	16km walk Zone #1	10km walk Zone #1 / 10km easy run	12km walk Zone #1 / 6km easy run	22km walk Zone #1	20km Hiking / 6km easy run	122km Total
7	15km walk Zone #1 / 6km easy run	12km walk Zone #1 / 5km easy run	15km walk Zone #1	12km walk Zone #1 / 10km easy run	12km walk Zone #1	25km walk Zone #1	20km Hiking / 8km easy run	140km Total
8	12km walk Zone #1 / 6km easy run	12km walk Zone #1 / 10km easy run	22km walk Zone #1	15km walk Zone #1	12km walk Zone #1 / 8km easy run	25km walk Zone #1	20km Hiking / 8km run	150km Total
9	15km walk Zone #1 / 6km easy run	12km walk Zone #1 / 6km easy run	25km walk Zone #1	15km walk Zone #1 / 8km easy run	12km walk Zone #1	20km walk Zone #1	10km run / Return from Altitude	130km Total

Phase II - Late Season Base Work for Olympic Level Athlete:

The Late Season Base Work phase lasts about 8 weeks. The goal during this phase is to increase your strength by walking some longer fartleks. These really help build your engine. We have also added a few shorter fartleks into the schedule. These serve three purposes. The first is just for the mental break from all of the longer training sessions that you have been walking. You will be amazed at how fast you can go with very little speedwork. The second is to get the kinks out of your legs and open up your stride a little bit as well as to have some fun. Finally, these allow you to test yourself so you don't go to the Millrose Games completely unprepared. The Millrose Games finishes up this phase and the #1 goal coming out of that race is to make sure you walk away injury

114

free. Walking on the steeply banked boards can be difficult and I wouldn't want you to go there and walk away injured. For myself, during each Olympic season, I have typically skipped the Millrose Games and instead chosen to not take the extra risk of walking a super fast mile. The choice is yours. If you choose to compete there, please make sure all precautions are taken so you walk away injury free. Here is the Late Season Base Phase for an Olympic level athlete:

Week	Monday	Tuesday	Wednesday	Thursday	Friday	Saturday	Sunday	Mileage
10 Rec Week	12km walk Zone #1 6km easy run	12km walk Zone #1	4km w-up Norwegian fartlek 2km c-d Zone # 3 8km easy run	18km walk Zone #1	12km walk Zone #1	15km walk Zone #1	20km walk Zone #1	120km Total
11	12km walk Zone #1 8km easy run	12km walk Zone #1	Fartlek 3km w-up 2 x 5km/1km 2km c-d Zone # 2 8km easy run	30km walk Zone #1	12km walk Zone #1	15km walk Zone #1 7km easy run	20km walk Zone #1	140km Total
12	12km walk Zone #1 8km easy run	15km walk Zone #1	Fartlek 3km w-up 3 x 5km/1km 2km c-d Zone # 2 8km easy run	Christmas Eve 12km run	Christmas DAY OFF	12km walk Zone #1	26km walk Zone #1	115km Total
13	12km walk Zone #1 6km easy run	Bohdan's Rhythm Workout 4km w-up 4 x 100, 200, 300, 400 with 100m easy walking between 2km c-d Zone #3/4 5km easy run	20km walk Zone #1	New Years Eve 12km walk Zone #1	New Years Day 5km walk Zone #1	3,000m Race to qualify for Indoor Nationals	20km walk Zone #1	100km Total

Week	Monday	Tuesday	Wednesday	Thursday	Friday	Saturday	Sunday	Mileage
14	12km walk Zone #1	LACTATE TEST 2km w-up 7 x 2km 2km c-d	22km walk Zone #1	15km walk Zone #1	12km walk Zone #1	3km w-up 12km TEMPO Zone #2 2km c-d	30km walk Zone #1	150km Total
		8km easy run		10km easy run		6km easy run		
15	12km walk Zone #1	15km walk Zone #1	25km walk Zone #1	12km walk Zone #1	12km walk Zone #1	Fartlek 3km w-up 3 x 5km/1km 2km c-d Zone # 2	30km walk Zone #1	160km Total
	8km easy run	8km easy run		10km easy run		6km easy run		
16	12km walk Zone #1	Fartlek 3km w-up 15 x 500/500 2km c-d Zone #3	20km walk Zone #1	OFF	12km walk Zone #1	Mexican Speedwork 3km w-up 4 x 1000, 800, 600, 400, 200 2km c-d 2 min rest Zone #3 / #4	25km walk Zone #1	135km Total
	8km easy run	5km easy run			8km easy run	8km easy run		
17	12km walk Zone #1	Speedwork 3km w-up 15 x 500m 2.5km c-d 90 seconds rest Zone #3	15km walk Zone #1	10km walk Zone #1	3km AM Pedestrian Walk	15km walk Zone #1	30km walk Zone #1	109km Total
		6km easy run			Millrose Games **1-Mile RACE**			

Phase III - In Season Racing for Olympic Level Athlete:

The In Season Racing phase for an Olympic-level athlete is going to be tough. There will be two harder sessions per week and it lasts for about 12 weeks. The goal during this phase will be to walk close to your 20km race pace, or your Zone #3, for many more kilometers than before. In order to be able to maintain the speeds necessary to obtain at least the minimum qualifications for the Olympics, you must be able to walk at 4:12/km for the men and at 4:53/km for the women. These are not easy, but if you can't walk these times for portions of your workouts, you are not ready to qualify for the Olympics.

As you will see, this phase includes a second altitude training camp soon after the U.S. Indoor Nationals. One month of total focus and dedication. This will be a great time to put all of your distractions out of your mind and focus on the task at hand – qualifying for the Olympic Games.

Coming down from altitude is a bit of a tricky task. Each person is going to adjust and adapt to returning to sea level differently. Typically an athlete needs to compete on either the 2nd, 3rd, or 4th day down from altitude, or they have to wait until after the 10th to 14th day. This is typically when, as Kjersti Plaetzer calls it, the "good days" come.

Your first 20km race of the season is scheduled for week #28. We have placed this race into the schedule since it is a typical weekend for when the World Cup Trials or America's Cup Trials are held.

Here is the In Season Racing phase for an Olympic level athlete:

Week	Monday	Tuesday	Wednesday	Thursday	Friday	Saturday	Sunday	Mileage
18	12km walk Zone #1	Fartlek 3km w-up 15 x 500/500 2km c-d Zone #3	20km walk Zone #1	15km walk Zone #1	12km walk Zone #1	2km w-up LACTATE TEST 7 x 2km 2km c-d	25km walk Zone #1	136km Total
	6km easy run	8km easy run						
19	12km walk Zone #1	Fartlek 3km w-up 10 x 1km/500 2km c-d Zone #3	20km walk Zone #1	15km walk Zone #1	12km walk Zone #1	Fartlek 3km w-up 7 x 2km/1km 2km c-d Zone #3	25km walk Zone #1	150km Total
	6km easy run	6km easy run		8km easy run		6km easy run		
20	12km walk Zone #1	Fartlek 3km w-up 12 x 1km/500 2km c-d Zone #3	20km walk Zone #1	15km walk Zone #1	12km walk Zone #1	Fartlek 3km w-up 3 or 4 x 4km/1km 2km c-d Zone #2 / #3	25km walk Zone #1	150km Total
	6km easy run	6km easy run		6km easy run				
21	12km walk Zone #1	Fartlek 3km w-up 18 x 500/500 2km c-d Zone #3	20km walk Zone #1	15km walk Zone #1	12km walk Zone #1	Speedwork 3km w-up 7 x 2km 2 min rest 2km c-d Zone #3	25km walk Zone #1	145km Total
		7km easy run		6km easy run		6km easy run		

Week	Monday	Tuesday	Wednesday	Thursday	Friday	Saturday	Sunday	Mileage
22	15km walk Zone #1	4km w-up Norwegian Fartlek 2km c-d Zone # 3 —— 8km easy run	20km walk Zone #1	OFF	12km walk Zone #1	Speedwork 3km w-up 12 x 1km 2km c-d Zone # 3 —— 7km easy run	15km walk Zone #1	110km Total
23	12km walk Zone #1	Speedwork 3km w-up 12 x 500m 2km c-d 90 sec rest Zone # 3 —— 6km easy run	12km walk Zone #1	8km walk Zone #1	6km walk Zone #1	USATF Indoor Nationals 5,000m	OFF	65km Total
24	8km walk Zone #1 —— 5km easy run	TRAVEL TO ALTITUDE —— 8km hiking	12km walk Zone #1 —— 8km easy run	18km walk Zone #1	12km walk Zone #1 —— 6km easy run	Fartlek 3km w-up 12 x 500/500 2km c-d Zone # 3 —— 6km easy run	20km walk Zone #1	120km Total
25	12km walk Zone #1	Fartlek 3km w-up 6 x 2km/1km 2km c-d Zone # 3 —— 6km easy run	20km walk Zone #1	15km walk Zone #1	12km walk Zone #1	Fartlek 3km w-up 12 x 1km/500 2km c-d Zone # 3 —— 6km easy run	25km walk Zone #1	141km Total
26	12km walk Zone #1	Fartlek 3km w-up 7 x 2km/1km 2km c-d Zone # 3 —— 5km easy run	22km walk Zone #1	12km walk Zone #1 —— 8km easy run	15km walk Zone #1	Fartlek 3km w-up 12 x 1km/500 2km c-d Zone # 3 —— 6km easy run	25km walk Zone #1	160km Total
27	12km walk Zone #1	Speedwork 3km w-up 8 x 2km 2km c-d 2 min rest Zone # 3 —— 6km easy run	20km walk Zone #1	15km walk Zone #1	12km walk Zone #1	Speedwork 3km w-up 12 x 1km 2km c-d 2 min rest Zone # 3 —— 6km easy run	15km walk Zone #1	124km Total
28	12km walk Zone #1	Speedwork 3km w-up 7 x 1km 6 x 500m 2km c-d Zone # 3 2 min rest	12km walk Zone #1 —— TRAVEL down from altitude to the race	12km walk Zone #1	6km walk Zone #1	20km RACE (World Cup Trials or America's Cup Trials)	6km easy run	88km Total
29 Rec. Week	OFF	12km walk Zone #1	15km walk Zone #1	12km walk Zone #1	Fartlek 3km w-up 12 x 500/500 2km c-d Zone # 3	18km walk Zone #1	15km walk Zone #1	95km Total

Phase IV - First Peak Season for an Olympic Level Athlete

The first peak of the season spans weeks 30 through 34. We chose this time period because it is a typical time when the IAAF World Cup is held as well as additional races in Europe. It is very important for you to remember if you want to be an Olympian you must compete against high level athletes in a conducive environment to walk fast times. If you don't have the time standard and you know a certain competition is sure to be slow due to the weather or being at altitude, it is probably a good idea to find another race to attend. Competing strong under tough conditions is very important to build your overall toughness, but not ideal for hitting a qualifying time.

Here is the First Peak Season phase for an Olympic level athlete:

Week	Monday	Tuesday	Wednesday	Thursday	Friday	Saturday	Sunday	Mileage
30	12km walk Zone #1	Speedwork 3km w-up 7 x 2km 2km c-d 2 min rest Zone #3 / 6 km easy run	20km walk Zone #1	12km walk Zone #1	Speedwork 3km w-up 12 x 1km 2 min rest 2km c-d Zone #3 / 6 km easy run	25km walk Zone #1	12km walk Zone #1	127km Total
31	Fartlek 3km w-up 15 x 500/500 2km c-d Zone # 3	18km walk Zone #1	12km walk Zone #1	Speedwork 3km w-up 7 x 2km 2km c-d 2 min rest Zone # 3	12km walk Zone #1	Fly to Europe 12km walk Zone #1	Arrive in Europe 8 km easy run	101km Total
32	12km walk Zone #1	Speedwork 3km w-up 10 x 500m 2km c-d 2 min rest Zone # 3	12km walk Zone #1	12km walk Zone #1	6km walk Zone #1	20km RACE	8km Hiking	85km Total
33	12km walk Zone #1 / 6 km hiking	18km walk Zone #1	4km w-up Norwegian Fartlek 2km c-d Zone # 3 / 6km easy run	15km walk Zone #1	12km walk Zone #1	Speedwork 3km w-up 7 x 2km 2km c-d Zone # 3	15km walk Zone #1	119km Total
34	12km walk Zone #1 / 6km easy run	15km walk Zone #1	Speedwork 4km w-up 10 x 500m with 90 seconds rest 2km c-d Zone # 3	15km walk Zone #1	10km walk with 10 x 1 min pickups in the middle	6km walk Zone #1	20km RACE	100km Total

Phase V - Second In Season Racing for Olympic Level Athletes

The Second In Season Racing phase lasts for 5-6 weeks, depending on when the Olympic Trials will be held. Most American athletes will peak for the Olympic Trails. The exception to this is if you are sure that when you cross the line at the trials you will have qualified for the team. This may happen if you are the only individual with a standard or one of no more than three "A" standard athletes in the race. Your season will end abruptly if you do not qualify, so take this race seriously.

In 2004 there were three of us, Kevin Eastler, John Nunn and myself, competing at the Olympic Trials who already achieved the "A" standard. Given the circumstances, we knew there was no one else who would be able to walk the "A" at the Trials, so it became a race for pride and prize money. The only way any one of us could not qualify to compete in Athens would have been if we were disqualified. None of us were going to take any extra risks, because the real focus on the day was to be an Olympian. The time we walked was irrelevant; the only thing that mattered was we finished the race. The three of us did what we had to do and we all qualified for the Olympic Games in Athens. Joy filled our faces, but sorrow would have filled out hearts if we were disqualified.

Here is the second In Season Racing phase for an Olympic level athlete:

Week	Monday	Tuesday	Wednesday	Thursday	Friday	Saturday	Sunday	Mileage
35	8km walk Zone #1	12km walk Zone #1	OFF	16km walk Zone #1	6km run	20km walk Zone #1	12km Hiking	74km Total
36	15km walk Zone #1	4km w-up Norwegian Fartlek 2km c-d Zone #3 / 6 km easy run	20km walk Zone #1	15km walk Zone #1	12km walk Zone #1	Speedwork 3km w-up 5 x 3km 2km c-d Zone #3 / 5 km easy run	25km walk Zone #1	135km Total
37	15km walk Zone #1	4km w-up Norwegian Fartlek 2km c-d Zone #3 / 8km easy run	20km walk Zone #1	15km walk Zone #1	12km walk Zone #1	Fartlek 3km w-up 4 x 4km/1km 2km c-d Zone #3 / 8km easy run	25km walk Zone #1	147km Total
38	12km walk Zone #1 / 7km easy run	Fartlek 3km w-up 12 x 1km/500 2km c-d Zone #3	15km walk Zone #1 / 8km easy run	12km walk Zone #1	12km walk Zone #1	Speedwork 3km w-up 3 x 5km 2 min rest 2km c-d Zone #3 / 6km easy run	25km walk Zone #1	140km Total
39	12km walk Zone #1 / 8km easy run	Speedwork 3km w-up 15 x 1km 2km c-d 2 min rest Zone #3 / 6km easy run	20km walk Zone #1	OFF	12km walk Zone #1	Speedwork 3km w-up 7 x 2km 2km c-d 2 min rest Zone # 3	22km walk Zone #1	125km Total

Phase VI - Second Peak Season for an Olympic Level Athlete

The Second Peak Season phase is a combination of In Season Racing phase and the Peak Season phase, as far as training goes. You must "peak" for the Olympic Trials, but you must make sure you

120

can maintain that peak for seven weeks. That is a tremendously difficult task. That is why this phase has a combination of the two.

After the Olympic Trials you need to recover properly before you lay your heart and soul on the line at the Olympic Games; the key is to use your head. You must race within your ability. As Coach Stephan Plaetzer has told me numerous times, "you must use the thing between your ears, don't just brush it." Kevin Eastler and I did just that in Athens when we moved up from 48th and 49th place leaving the Olympic stadium to 20th and 21st when we returned 1:25:00 later. You can exceed these performances if you use your head and race smart.

Here is the Second Peak Season phase for an Olympic level athlete:

Week	Monday	Tuesday	Wednesday	Thursday	Friday	Saturday	Sunday	Mileage
40	12km walk Zone #1	Speedwork 3km w-up 5km, 4km, 3km, 2km, 1km 2 min. rest 2km c-d Zone #2/#3 6km easy run	12km walk Zone #1	15km walk Zone #1	12km walk Zone #1	Speedwork 3km w-up 6 x 2km 2km c-d 2 min rest Zone #3	12km walk Zone #1	106km Total
41	12km walk Zone #1	3km w-up Norwegian Fartlek 2km c-d Zone #3	12km walk Zone #1	12km walk Zone #1	6km walk Zone #1	U.S. OLYMPIC TRIALS 20km RACE	8km easy run	91km Total
42 Rec. Week	10km easy run	12km walk Zone #1	15km walk Zone #1	15km walk Zone #1	4km w-up Norwegian Fartlek 3km c-d Zone #3	20km walk Zone #1	12km walk Zone #1	100km Total
43	12km walk Zone #1	Speedwork 3km w-up 3 x 3km 3 x 2km 3 x 1km 2 min rest 2km c-d Zone #3	20km walk Zone #1	8km walk Zone #1	12km walk Zone #1	Speedwork 3km w-up 20 x 500m 90 sec rest 2km c-d Zone #3 6 km easy run	20km walk Zone #1	116km Total
44	12km walk Zone #1	Speedwork 3km w-up 5km, 4km, 3km, 2km, 1km 2 min rest 2km c-d Zone #2/#3 5km easy run	12km walk Zone #1	20km walk Zone #1	12km walk Zone #1	Speedwork 3km w-up 8 x 2km 2 min rest 2km c-d Zone #3 5km easy run	18km walk Zone #1	125km Total

Week	Monday	Tuesday	Wednesday	Thursday	Friday	Saturday	Sunday	Mileage
45	12km walk Zone #1	Speedwork 3km w-up 12 x 1km 2km c-d 2 min rest Zone #3	18km walk Zone #1	15km walk Zone #1	12km walk Zone #1	Speedwork 3km w-up 6 x 2km 2km c-d 2 min rest Zone #3	15km walk Zone #1	104km Total
46	12km walk Zone #1	3km w-up Norwegian Fartlek 2km c-d Zone #3	15km walk Zone #1	10km walk Zone #1	10km walk Zone #1	8km walk Zone #1	**20km Olympic Games**	96km Total

Beyond the Olympics

One of the hardest things for many Olympians isn't their Olympic competition, but what happens after the end of the closing ceremonies. The Olympics are the pinnacle of athletic competition, something you worked toward and dreamt of for many years. Before the Games you were preparing, focusing and concentrating. During the Games you felt like the center of the world. Your family is fussing over you, the media is finally interested in you and you are living at the Olympic Village with over 10,000 other elite athletes from 200 countries. Your phone is ringing off the hook with people wishing you good luck, the media is begging for interviews, and your e-mail in-box gets filled up every day.

Then the Closing Ceremonies is completed with the symbolic extinguishing of the Olympic flame. A sadness overcomes you, as you bid farewell to your friends and make your way home. Upon returning, you are a normal person again. Your phone stops ringing and the media isn't begging for interviews. Instead, the bills are piling up and you realize that life is moving forward.

What do you do? You must find new goals. Upon the end of the 2004 Olympic Games, Curt Clausen went to Law School. At the end of the 2000 Olympic Games, Andrew Hermann went back to school for his MBA degree. It is imperative you find a new goal. If you are planning on trying to continue to be an elite athlete, focus on the next seasons IAAF World Championships. How are you going to improve upon your Olympic performance? What could you have done differently to assist you in having a better outcome? Find something you love to do and focus on it. That will be the key to your future.

TALES FROM THE TRACK – Andrew Hermann

Due to the distance there are many things an athlete can't control during a 50km. Therefore, being prepared mentally is just as important as being prepared physically. Going into the 2000 50km Olympic Trials I knew I was prepared physically and ready to go fast. Race day conditions however, dictated otherwise. With 50mph winds and pouring down rain, my mental perspective was that I was going to finish no matter what; I was going to race being in tuned with my body's feelings and thus adapt my pace accordingly; and I going to embrace the moment and race as hard as I could. This attitude enabled to me to adapt to extreme weather, constant changes in pace, and external factors that lead me to a 2nd place finish and qualifying for the Sydney Olympics.

Chapter Eight – Race Walking for Masters Athletes

With the exception of the Olympic level athletes, the Masters category might be the most competitive group in the country today. Starting at the age of 35, age groups exist for every five years. Competing as a Masters athlete is one of the most invigorating and life changing activities in which you can participate. Every five years you get to enter into a new age group and set a series of new goals. It will light a fire under you to try and break records and meet new challenges head on. The competitions, such as the USATF Masters Indoor Championships and the World Masters Championships, are some of the most populated events around the world each year. Some years over 10,000 athletes participant.

One of my former coaches, Bohdan Bulakowski, used to love to attend these events because it gave him a chance to see old friends and to compete against people at his level. The camaraderie these athletes seem to sustain is truly amazing, as many of them travel to and from competitions all over the world together.

Training and competing as a Master's athlete is a bit different than your younger counterparts for two reasons. The biggest issue is that while in general your training schedule is similar to younger athletes, you will need more recovery time between hard efforts. An extra day rest here or an extra recovery workout there is what is needed and required for you to excel at this level. This is especially hard for athletes who have race walked since they were younger. As athletes age they often try to repeat the formula they used for success in the past. Unfortunately, if older walkers try to train as they did when they were younger they may excel initially, but over time, consistency is difficult to maintain and one's propensity to get injured skyrockets. Instead, you must give the body time to rebuild when you break it down through hard workouts.

Depending on your availability, your level of commitment, and of course, your ability to stay injury free, you are able to train five or six days a week, but you must give yourself at least two or three days of recovery time in between your harder sessions during the In Season Racing and Peak Season phases. Any less time and you won't recover properly and risk injury or burn out. Time and time again athletes have tried to buck this system and skip their recovery by trying to squeeze in another hard day and the end result is consistent failure. Don't let this happen to you. Always focus on good recovery.

The second issue which separates Masters athletes from their young peers is they want to peak for many different races. While you cannot continually peak, the schedule we devised for you allows you to have a mini-peak for indoors and a bigger peak outdoors.

Getting Started

Masters athletes come in three flavors: those who were previously sedentary, those who were active in other sports, and those who race walked in their younger years. The first two groups may wish to simply walk a 5km at least three times a week before starting our program. These walks should all be done at an easy Zone #1 pace. This will give you time to adapt to the stress of a new form of exercise. The third group can step right into our program.

Developing a Schedule for Masters Race Walkers

Masters athletes present a unique problem for a coach trying to create a coherent well-thought-out training plan. Masters athletes rarely have a single goal. Elite athletes make it easy; they want to qualify for the Olympics. This allows a coach to develop a systematic multi-year plan. Masters athletes often want to rack up as many age-group medals/records as they can at varied distances at races spread out geographically and chronologically.

For elite Masters race walkers the first big races of the season are in March with the USATF Masters Indoor Championship (3,000m) and the World Masters Indoor Championships (3,000m and 10km) which occur every other year. These are followed by a series of races in late July and August at the USATF Outdoor Masters Championships (5,000m and 10km) as well as the World Masters Outdoor Championships (5,000m, 10km, 20km), which are contested every other year opposite the World Masters Indoor Championships. Given this diversity of goals, we suggest training primarily for a 10km and stepping down to the shorter races. If your main goal is the 20km, you'll want to take our advice and add distance to the longer days as well as increase the distance and number of intervals of the harder efforts.

The TEAMS system of training is periodic and typically has four main phases; the Youth, High School and Collegiate athletes utilize a single peak season. However, the Olympic Level athletes, we utilized a dual peak season whereby the athletes could peak in May and then again in July/August. Similarly, for the Master's athletes, we detail a double peak season; one for the indoor season, March, and the second for the outdoor championship races, around July/August. After the initial peak in March, we regroup with a recovery period before building back up with another In Season Racing phase. This leads to a final more intense peak phase. Therefore, a Masters athlete program is comprised of seven phases. Utilizing the TEAMS system, you should be able to adapt the training to your own needs and schedule and excel at the same time. Find a balance and your life will be in sync.

Next is a sample training schedule for a Masters athlete preparing for a 10km race with the appropriate tapers in place to step down for the shorter distances as needed. Also, as previously stated, if you want to focus on a 20km as your main goal, simply increase the long days and hard workouts in distance slightly or in the number of repetitions.

Phase I - Early Season Base Work for Masters Race Walkers

The Early Season Base Work phase for Masters race walkers is similar to the schedules of their more youthful brethren. The template is similar, but the Masters schedule has an additional day of recovery time so vital to Masters walkers. Less experienced walkers, as well as walkers over 60, will probably want to take two days off a week. Younger experienced walkers can add the extra day of Zone #1 walking. This gives your body the best recovery possible as we start to move forward with the season. Pushing too much too soon is only going to risk peaking early and increasing your risk for an injury. In addition, Masters walkers should try to perform technique drills every day they race walk. Masters walkers typically suffer from a smaller range of motion. How many of you claim that you are totally inflexible? Therefore, combat this head-on with technique drills before workouts and a healthy amount of stretching afterward.

Pick the starting date by working backward from your final goal race. We have chosen to start your schedule in October so you'll peak appropriately for many of the big races. Also, note you need to have some form of active rest if you previously finished a hard training season. Many Masters walkers want to roll from one season to another. Your body needs time to heal and rebuild from the previous season before starting over. Also note, if you are an experienced walker you could add more distance to your Zone #1 workouts, but do not increase the intensity. If the idea of hiking isn't appealing, you may replace it with Zone #1 work. However, don't discount the benefits of a good hike to build your capillary system! We have also added some 1-minute pickups after week #3, just to get your legs moving and to help out from any boredom that might be happening during the base training period.

Note that the total weekly mileage shown in the charts is the maximum weekly mileage. If you take the additional day off, your actual total weekly mileage will be lower.

Here is the Early Season Base Work phase for a Masters race walkers:

Week	Monday	Tuesday	Wednesday	Thursday	Friday	Saturday	Sunday	Mileage
1	5km walk Zone #1	OFF	5km walk Zone #1	5km walk Zone #1	OFF	8km walk Zone #1	10km hiking	33km total
2	6km walk Zone #1	OFF	6km walk Zone #1	5km walk Zone #1	OFF	10km walk Zone #1	12km hiking	39km Total
3	7km walk Zone #1	OFF or 5km walk Zone #1	7km walk Zone #1	5km walk Zone #1	OFF	10km walk Zone #1	12km hiking	46km total
4	5km walk Zone #1	OFF or 5km walk Zone #1	10km Hiking	5km walk Zone #1 with 5 x 1 min Pickups in the middle	OFF	12km walk Zone #1	14km Hiking	51km Total
5	6km walk Zone #1	OFF or 5km walk Zone #1	10km walk Zone #1	8km walk Zone #1	OFF	10km walk Zone #1	15km hiking	54km Total
6 Rec. Week	6km walk Zone #1	OFF or 5km walk Zone #1	6km walk Zone #1	8km walk Zone #1	OFF	8km walk Zone #1	10km hiking	43km Total

Phase II - Late Season Base Work phase for Masters Race Walkers

The Late Season Base Work phase for Masters race walkers prepares you for what is to come. You will notice that you still have off one to two days a week, but we have dropped the hiking and replaced it with Zone #1 walking. As always, you should do your technique/mobility drills five or six times per week.

The Late Season Base Work phase typically lasts seven weeks spanning December and January. It increases the distance of many of the workouts as well as including a new workout, a longer fartlek. A longer fartlek, in this phase, is a walk where the fast portions of the workout are walked at Zone #2 pace and the slower portions are walked at Zone #1 pace. The intervals will vary from 2km "fast" and 1km "slow" to as long as 4km "fast" and 1km "slow".

Note, you still want to walk your Zone #1 workouts at the appropriate pace.

Here is a schedule for the Late Season Base Work phase for Masters race walkers:

Week	Monday	Tuesday	Wednesday	Thursday	Friday	Saturday	Sunday	Mileage
7	6km walk Zone #1	OFF or 5km walk Zone #1	7km walk Zone #1	2km w-up LACTATE TEST 5 x 2km 2km c-d	OFF	6km walk Zone #1	10km walk Zone #1	48 km total
8	6km walk Zone #1	OFF or 5km walk Zone #1	8km walk Zone #1	Fartlek 2km w-up 2 x 2km/2km Zone # 2	OFF	7km walk Zone #1	12km Zone #1	48km total
9	7km walk Zone #1	OFF or 5km walk Zone #1	8km walk Zone #1	Fartlek 2km w-up 3 x 2km/1km Zone # 2 2km c-d	OFF	8km walk Zone #1	12km Zone #1	53km total
10	8km walk Zone #1	OFF or 5km walk Zone #1	8km walk Zone #1	Fartlek 2km w-up 2 x 3km/1km Zone # 2 2km c-d	OFF	8km walk Zone #1	14km Zone #1	55km Total
11	8km walk Zone #1	OFF or 5km walk Zone #1	8km walk Zone #1	Fartlek 2km w-up 2 x 3km/1km Zone # 2 2km c-d	OFF	8km walk Zone #1	15km Zone #1	56km Total

126

Week	Monday	Tuesday	Wednesday	Thursday	Friday	Saturday	Sunday	Mileage
12	8km walk Zone #1	OFF or 5km walk Zone #1	8km walk Zone #1	Fartlek 2km w-up 2 x 4km/1km Zone #2 2km c-d	OFF	8km walk Zone #1	15km Zone #1	58km Total
13 Rec. Week	OFF or 6km walk Zone #1	8km walk Zone #1	8km walk Zone #1	OFF	6km walk Zone #1	8km walk Zone #1	12km walk Zone #1	48km Total

Phase III - First In Season Racing for Masters Race Walkers

The third phase lasts nine weeks and gets you ready for your first set of goals, the indoor championships. The goal of this phase is to push your lactate threshold higher while still walking enough mileage to maintain your strength through the end of the season. While we increase the intensity, note we still offer up to two days off per week. Make sure you rest properly. Remember, your goal is to peak twice, so make sure you are getting enough rest.

Note, the First In Season Racing phase for Masters race walkers includes two races:

Week	Monday	Tuesday	Wednesday	Thursday	Friday	Saturday	Sunday	Mileage
14	OFF or 6km walk Zone #1	Fartlek 2km w-up 3 x 2km/1km 2km c-d Zone # 3	10km walk Zone #1	OFF	6km walk Zone #1	Fartlek 3km w-up 6 x 500/500 2km c-d Zone #3	12km walk Zone #1	58km Total
15	OFF or 8km walk Zone #1	Fartlek 2km w-up 3 x 2km/1km 2k c-d Zone # 3	11km walk Zone #1	OFF	6km walk Zone #1	Fartlek 3km w-up 8 x 500/500 2km c-d Zone #3	14km walk Zone #1	65km Total
16	OFF or 10km walk Zone #1	Fartlek 2km w-up 5 x 1km/500m 2km c-d Zone #3	12km walk Zone #1	OFF	6km walk Zone #1	Rhythm 3km w-up 4 x 100, 200, 300, 400m w/ 100m between 2 km c-d Zone #4	16km walk Zone #1	66km Total
17 Rec. Week	OFF or 5km walk Zone #1	8km walk Zone #1	Speedwork 3km w-up 6 x 1000m 3 min rest 2km c-d Zone #3	OFF	8km walk Zone #1	15km walk Zone #1	OFF	47km Total

Week	Monday	Tuesday	Wednesday	Thursday	Friday	Saturday	Sunday	Mileage
18	OFF or 8km walk Zone #1	Fartlek 2km w-up 5 x 1km/500m 2km c-d Zone #3	10km walk Zone #1	OFF	6km walk Zone #1	3km w-up Mexican Speedwork 2 x 1000, 800, 600, 400, 200 Zone #3/4 2 min rest 2km c-d Zone #3	15km walk Zone #1	61km Total
19	OFF or 6km walk Zone #1	Speedwork 2 km w-up 6 x 400m Zone #3 90 sec rest 2km c-d	8km walk Zone #1	OFF	2-5km walk Zone #1	2km w-up **1-Mile or 3,000m RACE** 2km c-d	12km walk Zone #1	44km Total
20	6km walk Zone #1	OFF	Fartlek 2km w-up 8 x 500/500 2km c-d Zone #3	6km walk Zone #1	6km walk Zone #1	3km w-up Mexican Speedwork 2 x 1000, 800, 600, 400, 200 2 min rest 2km c-d Zone # 3	12km walk Zone #1	53km Total
21	OFF or 6km walk Zone #1	Speedwork 2 km w-up 6 x 400m Zone #3 90 sec rest 2km c-d	10km walk Zone #1	OFF	6km walk Zone #1	2-5km walk Zone #1	**3,000m or 5,000 Race**	36km Total
22 Rec. Week	6km walk Zone #1	OFF	8km walk Zone #1	6km walk Zone #1	Fartlek 3km w-up 6 x 500/500 2km c-d Zone #3	12km walk Zone #1	OFF	43km Total

As you can see, racing greatly effects your abililty to train. This is why trying to peak twice is so difficult. Don't worry though. Given the length of the season and our focus on recovery, if you are patient and follow our guidelines, you will recover from your races and be ready to peak again later in the season.

Phase IV - First Peak Season for Masters Race Walkers

The First Peak Season Phase for Masters race walkers occurs during for the indoor season. Since the World Masters Indoor Championships are held every other year, we have chosen to provide the more complicated year for you to balance your training. If you are competing in a year without it, simply modify the schedule to reflect one less race.

Here is the first Peak Season phase for Masters race walkers:

Week	Monday	Tuesday	Wednesday	Thursday	Friday	Saturday	Sunday	Mileage
23	8km walk Zone #1 Or OFF	Speedwork 3km w-up 3km, 2km, 1km 2km c-d 3:00 rest Zone #3/#4	10km walk Zone #1	OFF	6km walk Zone #1	3km w-up Mexican Speedwork 2 x 1000, 800, 600, 400, 200 2 min rest 2km c-d Zone #3/#4	12km walk Zone #1	58km Total
24	8km walk Zone #1 Or OFF	Speedwork 3km w-up 4 x 1km 4 x 500m 2:30 rest 2km c-d Zone # 3	8km walk Zone #1	OFF	Speedwork 3km w-up 8 x 500m 2 min rest 2km c-d Zone # 3	8km walk Zone #1	8km walk Zone #1	52km Total
25	OFF or 5km walk Zone #1	3km to 5km walk Zone #1	3,000m RACE WMA Indoor Championships	OFF or 3km walk Zone #1	10km RACE WMA Indoor Championships	OFF	6km walk Zone #1	40km Total
26 Rec. Week	8km walk Zone #1 or OFF	10km walk Zone #1	8km walk Zone #1	OFF	6km walk Zone #1	3km w-up Mexican Speedwork 2 x 1000, 800, 600, 400, 200 2 min rest 2km c-d Zone # 4	10km walk Zone #1	43km Total
27	OFF	8km walk Zone #1	Speedwork 3km w-up 6 x 500m 2 min rest 2km c-d Zone # 3	OFF	6km walk Zone #1	3km to 5km walk Zone #1	3,000m RACE USATF Masters Indoor Nationals	34km Total

Recovery for the First Peak Season for Masters Athletes

Because a Masters walker is likely to desire two peaks during the year, we added an additional phase not included in the other training schedules. This divergence from our standard four phase progression is a return to the template for late season base building for a total duration of four weeks. This temporarily tones down your training to recover and thus allow a bigger and faster peak in July and August. This is accomplished by repeating the late season base phase for about four weeks in April.

Week	Monday	Tuesday	Wednesday	Thursday	Friday	Saturday	Sunday	Mileage
28 Rec. Week	6km walk Zone #1	OFF	6km walk Zone #1	8km walk Zone #1	OFF	8km walk Zone #1	10km hiking	38km Total
29 Rec. Week	8km walk Zone #1	OFF	8km walk Zone #1	10km walk Zone #1	OFF	10km walk Zone #1	10km hiking	46km Total
30 Rec. Week	10km walk Zone #1	OFF	8km walk Zone #1	10km walk Zone #1	OFF	Fartlek 3km w-up 8 x 500/500 2km c-d Zone #3	10km Zone #1	51km Total
31 Rec. Week	12km walk Zone #1	OFF	10km walk Zone #1	10km walk Zone #1	OFF	Fartlek 3km w-up 8 x 500/500 2km c-d Zone #3	12km walk Zone #1	57km Total

Phase V - Second In Season Racing for Masters Race Walkers

After a proper recovery, you are ready to build your engine again for the months of May and June. Notice that the intervals are longer than during the indoor In Season Racing phase. Having built a solid base you are now ready for more intense training. This becomes especially necessary as you lengthen the distance of your races to 10km or even 20km.

Here is the Second In Season Racing phase for Masters race walkers:

Week	Monday	Tuesday	Wednesday	Thursday	Friday	Saturday	Sunday	Mileage
32	8km walk Zone #1 Or OFF	Fartlek 3km w-up 6 x 1km/500m 2k c-d Zone #3	12km walk Zone #1	OFF	6km walk Zone #1	3km w-up Mexican Speedwork 2 x 1000, 800, 600, 400, 200 2 min rest 2km c-d Zone #4	12km walk Zone #1	63km Total
33	OFF or 8km walk Zone #1	LACTATE TEST 2km w-up 6 x 2km 2km c-d	10km walk Zone #1	OFF	6km walk Zone #1	Fartlek 3km w-up 10 x 500/500 2km c-d Zone # 3	15km walk Zone #1	70km Total
34 Rec. Week	OFF	6km walk Zone #1	8km walk Zone #1	OFF	6km walk Zone #1	Speedwork 3km w-up 12 x 400m 2km c-d Zone # 4	12km walk Zone #1	42km Total

130

Week	Monday	Tuesday	Wednesday	Thursday	Friday	Saturday	Sunday	Mileage
35	OFF or 8km walk Zone #1	Spanish Fartlek 3km w-up 8 x 800m/400m 2km c-d Zone # 3	12km walk Zone #1	OFF	6km walk Zone #1	Bohdan's Rhythm Workout 3km w-up 4 x 100, 200, 300, 400 with 100m easy between 2km c-d Zone # 4	15km walk Zone #1	67km Total
36	OFF or 8km walk Zone #1	Fartlek 3km w-up 4 x 2km/1km 2km c-d Zone # 3	10km walk Zone #1	OFF	6km walk Zone #1	Fartlek 3km w-up 8 x 500/500 2km c-d Zone # 3	16km walk Zone #1	70km Total
37	OFF or 8km walk Zone #1	Fartlek 3km w-up 4 x 2km/1km 2km c-d Zone # 3	10km walk Zone #1	OFF	6km walk Zone #1	Fartlek 3km w-up 8 x 500/500 2km c-d Zone # 3	18km walk Zone #1	72km Total
38	OFF or 8km walk Zone #1	Fartlek 2km w-up 6 x 1km/500m 2km c-d Zone # 3	10km walk Zone #1	OFF	6km walk Zone #1	Fartlek 3km w-up 10 x 500/500 2km c-d Zone # 3	18km walk Zone #1	70km Total
39 Rec. Week	OFF	6km walk Zone #1	8km walk Zone #1	OFF	6km walk Zone #1	Speedwork 3km w-up 12 x 500m 2km c-d 2 min rest Zone #4	12km walk Zone #1	43km Total

Phase VI - Second Peak Season for Masters Race Walkers

As you all know, you can't peak for every race at every distance. This schedule is set up for you to peak when it counts – at the USATF Masters Outdoor Championships and the World Masters Outdoor Championships. Make sure you are getting enough recovery and staying well hydrated as the weather will undoubtedly be getting warmer during this time.

Here is the second Peak Season for Masters race walkers:

Week	Monday	Tuesday	Wednesday	Thursday	Friday	Saturday	Sunday	Mileage
40	OFF or 8km walk Zone #1	Speedwork 3km w-up 4 x 2km 2km c-d 2:30 rest Zone # 3	10km walk Zone #1	OFF	6km walk Zone #1	Mexican Speedwork 3km w-up 2 x 1000, 800, 600, 400, 200 2 min rest 2km c-d Zone # 4	15km walk Zone #1	63km Total
41	OFF or 8km walk Zone #1	Speedwork 3km w-up 6 x 1km 2km c-d 2 min rest Zone # 3	10km walk Zone #1	OFF	6km walk Zone #1	Speedwork 3km w-up 8 x 500m 2 min rest 2km c-d Zone # 3	10km walk Zone #1	54km Total
42	OFF or 6km walk Zone #1	6km walk Zone #1 with 6 x 1-min pickups	5km walk Zone #1	3km to 5km walk Zone #1	5,000m RACE	OFF or 3km to 5km walk Zone #1	10km Race	50km Total
43 Rec. Week	OFF	5km walk Zone #1	6km walk Zone #1	OFF	8km walk Zone #1	Speedwork 3km w-up 6 x 800m 2km c-d Zone # 3	15km walk Zone #1	44km Total
44	OFF or 6km walk Zone #1	Speedwork 3km w-up 8 x 1km 2km c-d 2 min rest Zone # 3	10km walk Zone #1	OFF	8km walk Zone #1	Mexican Speedwork 3km –up 2 x 1000, 800, 600, 400, 200 2 min rest 2km c-d Zone # 4	12km walk Zone #1	60km Total
45	OFF or 8km walk Zone #1	Speedwork 3km w-up 8 x 400m 2km c-d 2 min rest Zone # 4	8km walk Zone #1	OFF	5km walk Zone #1	5,000m Race	OFF or 4km walk Zone #1	43km Total
46	10km Race	OFF or 4km walk Zone #1	4km walk Zone #1	20km Race	OFF	6km walk Zone #1	OFF	52km Total

Chapter Nine – Race Walking a Marathon

While the marathon isn't a race walking typical distance contested as part of track and field in any of the major international competitions, many walkers gravitate to the challenge of completing the 26.2-mile event. Those lured into trying to finish a marathon or race one for time are mostly beginner walkers, as elite walkers usually only participate in a marathon as a training session for the 50km. Therefore, our training schedule is designed for beginner and early intermediate walkers.

Since marathons are primarily marked by miles instead of kilometers, we've modified our training schedule format to measure distances in miles. Both the beginner and intermediate programs work on a monthly cycle where your mileage/intensity increases for three weeks followed by a week of recovery to allow the body to build upon the work you have completed. The next cycle begins with a slight decrease in mileage from the third week of the previous cycle and then builds to a higher level in the following cycle.

Developing a Marathon Schedule for Beginner Race Walkers

Our schedule to train a beginning walker to complete a marathon is a departure from the traditional multi-phase approach shown in the rest of the text. We do this because beginning walkers are not racing the marathon but usually just trying to complete the distance in some vague time goal; like six, seven, or eight hours. As such, training is simply a matter of a conservative progression of distance walks which adapt the body to the stresses of walking 26.2 miles continuously.

Before starting our beginner marathon program, you should be comfortable walking five miles three to five days per week. If you are not ready to walk that much, then build up to it before starting our program.

The key to a beginner marathon training program is the long day. While our schedule shows the long day on Sunday, you can move it to any other day of the week so that it fits your personal schedule as long as you ensure adequate recovery time between it and the other harder days. In addition, there is a second medium distance day. This day can also be moved around, but is ideally placed two or three days from the long day. For illustrative purposes, we've included it on Thursday. Both the long and medium distance days are walked at a Zone #1 pace, which is basically your marathon race pace. If you've trained at race pace for over five months, when you finally get to the marathon, you'll know exactly how fast to go. Additionally, we've thrown in some shorter fartleks to keep the legs and mind fresh. These are not like the fartleks in the rest of the book. Instead, they are shorter fartleks with only the intensity of a Zone #2 walk and are geared for beginner marathoners to get a sense of a quicker pace. We do not prescribe doing longer fartleks, more repetitions, or quicker intensity as the increase in weekly distance is enough stress on your body.

Again, try to have an easy- or off-day in between any fartlek workout or distance day. For our schedule we've placed the fartlek workout on Tuesdays, when the week includes one, to break up the longer workouts. The rest of the days of the schedule are easy Zone #1 walks or days off. We've set our schedule for five days of walking per week, as most beginners will not dedicate six days. If you wish to add a sixth day, simply replace one of the off-days with a five-mile Zone #1 walk.

Given the schedule we've presented you can take your days off on either Monday, Wednesday, or Friday. We've selected Wednesday and Friday as the stresses of work tend to tire you out as the week goes on and you may be less likely to get out the door later in the week. However, if your schedule is better suited to taking your days off on Monday and Friday, feel free to change the days around.

The maximum distance walked in the schedule is 20 miles. Do not walk more than this as you may not recover in time for the marathon. Walking a 20-miler takes a lot out of the body. The three weeks provided from your 20-miler until your marathon are necessary. This enables the body to absorb all of the work you've accomplished and fully recover so you are fresh for the marathon on race day. Walking 20 miles at the proper Zone #1 pace makes a huge deposit in your training bank and if you rest properly, you'll be able to withdraw it with interest on race day. Most walkers who can complete the 20 mile workout are physically fit enough to complete a marathon as the adrenalin of race day as well as the weeks of tapering will carry you through the last 6.2 miles.

If you don't walk 5 days a week, but choose to walk three or four days a week by taking off the shorter days, you probably will still be able to complete the marathon. However, doing so will be far less comfortable and your recovery will be significantly more difficult. Therefore, try to walk five days per week if your schedule permits.

Month One - Beginner Marathon Training

The first month of training is a simple progression of mileage where the distance workout on Sunday gets longer each week.

Week	Monday	Tuesday	Wednesday	Thursday	Friday	Saturday	Sunday	Mileage
1	5 miles	5 miles	OFF	6 miles	OFF	5 miles	8 miles	29 miles
2	5 miles	5 miles	OFF	6 miles	OFF	5 miles	10 miles	31 miles
3	5 miles	5 miles	OFF	6 miles	OFF	5 miles	12 miles	33 miles
4	OFF	5 miles	OFF	5 miles	OFF	5 miles	6 miles	21 miles

Month Two - Beginner Marathon Training

The second month of training adds two fartlek workouts to keep the legs fresh. The fartleks have an equal amount of distance walked in Zone #1 and Zone #2. This will give your body plenty of time to recover from the higher intensity intervals. You may feel your shins are a little sore after doing them, so make sure you cool down properly with shin and calf stretches to reduce the strain the higher intensity may cause.

Week	Monday	Tuesday	Wednesday	Thursday	Friday	Saturday	Sunday	Mileage
5	5 miles	Fartlek 2 mile w-up 8 x 1/4 mile Zone #2 1/4 mile Zone #1 1 mile c-d	OFF	7 miles	OFF	5 miles	10 miles	32 miles
6	5 miles	5 miles	OFF	7 miles	OFF	5 miles	12 miles	34 miles
7	5 miles	Fartlek 2 mile w-up 4 x 1/2 mile Zone #2 1/2 mile Zone #1 1 mile c-d	OFF	7 miles	OFF	5 miles	14 miles	36 miles
8 Rec. Week	OFF	5 miles	OFF	5 miles	OFF	5 miles	8 miles	23 miles

Month Three - Beginning Marathon Training

During the third month, your distance continues to grow and your fartleks become more challenging. Now, instead of walking an equal distance in Zone #1 and Zone #2, the Zone #2 intervals of the fartlek are twice as far as the Zone #1 portions.

Week	Monday	Tuesday	Wednesday	Thursday	Friday	Saturday	Sunday	Mileage
9	5 miles	Fartlek 2 mile w-up 4 x 1/2 mile Zone #2 1/4 mile Zone #1 1 mile c-d	OFF	8 miles	OFF	5 miles	12 miles	36 miles
10	5 miles	6 miles	OFF	8 miles	OFF	5 miles	14 miles	38 miles
11	5 miles	Fartlek 2 mile w-up 6 x 1/2 mile Zone #2 1/4 mile Zone #1 1 mile c-d	OFF	8 miles	OFF	5 miles	16 miles	41.5 miles
12 Rec. Week	OFF	5 miles	OFF	5 miles	OFF	5 miles	10 miles	25 miles

Month Four - Beginning Marathon Training

During this month, both your overall distance and the intervals of the fartlek increase.

Week	Monday	Tuesday	Wednesday	Thursday	Friday	Saturday	Sunday	Mileage
13	6 miles	Fartlek 2 mile w-up 3 x 1 mile Zone #2 1/2 mile Zone #1 1 mile c-d	OFF	9 miles	OFF	6 miles	14 miles	42.5 miles
14	6 miles	7 miles	OFF	9 miles	OFF	6 miles	16 miles	44 miles
15	6 miles	Fartlek 2 mile w-up 3 x 1 mile Zone #2 1/4 mile Zone #1 1 mile c-d	OFF	9 miles	OFF	6 miles	18 miles	46.5 miles
16 Rec. Week	OFF	5 miles	OFF	5 miles	OFF	5 miles	10 miles	25 miles

Month Five - Beginning Marathon Training

The fifth month is really the last month of your training. After this month, it's all about recovery for the marathon. Many walkers struggle fitting the longer walks into their life schedule. Try to plan ahead and leave yourself time during this month. Walking the 16, 18, and 20 milers is the best preparation for your marathon, so set yourself up for success by getting in your key workouts.

Week	Monday	Tuesday	Wednesday	Thursday	Friday	Saturday	Sunday	Mileage
17	7 miles	Fartlek 2 mile w-up 8 x 1/2 mile Zone #2 1/4 mile Zone #1 1 mile c-d	OFF	10 miles	OFF	6 miles	16 miles	48 miles
18	7 miles	7 miles	OFF	10 miles	OFF	6 miles	18 miles	48 miles
19	7 miles	Fartlek 2 mile w-up 10 x 1/4 mile Zone #2 1/4 mile Zone #1 1 mile c-d	OFF	10 mlies	OFF	6 miles	20 miles	51 miles
20 Rec. Week	OFF	5 miles	OFF	5 miles	OFF	5 miles	10 miles	25 miles

Taper - Beginning Marathon Training

The work is all done now. For the last two weeks, the most important aspect of your training is rest. It's too late to go out and make up the mileage. You need to enter your marathon well rested and ready to walk.

Week	Monday	Tuesday	Wednesday	Thursday	Friday	Saturday	Sunday	Mileage
21	7 miles	Fartlek 2 mile w-up 6 x 1/2 mile Zone # 2 1/4 mile Zone #1 1 mile c/d	OFF	5 miles	OFF	5 miles	10 miles	34.5 miles
22	5 miles	OFF	5 miles	3 miles	OFF	2 miles	Marathon Day	41 miles

Developing a Marathon Schedule for Intermediate Race Walkers

Our schedule to train an intermediate walker to complete a marathon is similar to that of the beginner walker in that it still is primarily based on a progression of distance walks adapting the body to the stresses of walking 26.2 miles. However, the intermediate walker starts with more weekly mileage, as well as builds to longer and more intense fartlek workouts. This enables someone following this program not only to walk a faster marathon, but to be capable of stepping down to shorter distances like a 20km or half marathon and race them as well.

Before starting our intermediate marathon program, you should be comfortable walking 10 miles in a single workout and have walked up to 40 miles in a week. If you are not ready to walk that much distance, then build up to it before starting our program.

Again the key to the program is the distance day, but walking the fartleks properly is the way to increased speed and ultimately your marathon pace. Like the beginner schedule, it is set up to walk five days per week. As an intermediate marathoner you should not try to train on less than five days. It's probably better to get in 6 days a week of training by adding 5-7 miles of Zone #1 walking on either Wednesday or Friday, but as we know time is short and marathon training takes up a lot of it. So use your judgment on whether you want to walk five or six days a week.

Month One - Intermediate Marathon Training

The first month of training is a simple progression of mileage where the distance workout on Sunday gets longer each week. In addition, the other Zone #1 walks increase in length as well.

Week	Monday	Tuesday	Wednesday	Thursday	Friday	Saturday	Sunday	Mileage
1	5 miles	5 miles	OFF	8 miles	OFF	5 miles	10 miles	33 miles
2	6 miles	5 miles	OFF	8 miles	OFF	6 miles	12 miles	37 miles
3	7 miles	6 miles	OFF	8 miles	OFF	7 miles	14 miles	42 miles
4	OFF	6 miles	OFF	6 miles	OFF	6 miles	7 miles	25 miles

Month Two - Intermediate Marathon Training

The second month of the schedule continues the mileage build up, while adding a longer fartlek every other week. The fartleks are just a taste of the harder workouts to come. It is important not to do them too fast. So, keep the harder portions of the fartlek to the **lower end** of Zone #3. These are not designed for sprinting a fast 5km, but to help you improve your pace for the marathon.

Week	Monday	Tuesday	Wednesday	Thursday	Friday	Saturday	Sunday	Mileage
5	7 miles	Fartlek 2 mile w-up 3 x 1 mile Zone #3 1/2 mile Zone #1 1 mile c-d	OFF	9 miles	OFF	7 miles	12 miles	41.5 miles
6	7 miles	7 miles	OFF	9 miles	OFF	7 miles	14 miles	44 miles
7	7 miles	Fartlek 2 mile w-up 5 x 3/4 mile Zone #3 1/4 mile Zone #1 1 mile c-d	OFF	9 miles	OFF	7 miles	16 miles	47 miles
8 Rec. Week	OFF	6 miles	OFF	6 miles	OFF	6 miles	8 miles	24 miles

Month Three - Intermediate Marathon Training

By your third month, you come close to reaching your maximum mileage on your longest walks as well as the number of higher intensity workouts in the form of fartleks. During this month you walk at least one fartlek every week and add two shorter fartleks to work on your leg speed. The shorter fartleks may be walked slightly faster than the longer ones during the intervals.

Week	Monday	Tuesday	Wednesday	Thursday	Friday	Saturday	Sunday	Mileage
9	7miles	Fartlek 2 mile w-up 2 x 1 1/2 miles Zone # 3 1/2 mile Zone #1 1 mile c-d	OFF	9 miles	OFF	Fartlek 2 mile w-up 6 x 1/2 mile Zone # 3 1/4 mile Zone #1 1 mile c-d	14 miles	44.5 miles

Week	Monday	Tuesday	Wednesday	Thursday	Friday	Saturday	Sunday	Mileage
10	7 miles	Fartlek 2 mile w-up 3 x 1 mile Zone #3 1/2 mile Zone #1 1 mile c-d	OFF	9 miles	OFF	7 miles	16 miles	46.5 miles
11	7 miles	Fartlek 2 mile w-up 4 x 3/4 mile Zone #3 1/4 mile Zone #1 1 mile c-d	OFF	9 miles	OFF	Fartlek 2 mile w-up 6 x 1/2 mile Zone # 3 1/4 mile Zone #1 1 mile c-d	18 miles	48.5 miles
12 Rec. Week	OFF	5 miles	OFF	5 miles	OFF	5 miles	10 miles	25 miles

Month Four - Intermediate Marathon Training

Unlike the beginner schedule, you will be walking 20 miles twice. The first time is during the fourth month. In addition, the total distance walked at harder effort is increased during the fartleks. Pay attention to your pacing on the longer walks. It's always better to start off slowly and increase than to blast out hard and come back depleted. **You should never feel wiped out after your long walks. If you do, you are walking at too quick of a pace and need to slow down.**

Week	Monday	Tuesday	Wednesday	Thursday	Friday	Saturday	Sunday	Mileage
13	7 miles	Fartlek 2 mile w-up 2 x 1 1/2 miles Zone # 3 1/2 mile Zone #1 1 mile c-d	OFF	10 miles	OFF	Fartlek 2 mile w-up 6 x 1/2 mile Zone # 3 1/4 mile Zone #1 1 mile c-d	16 miles	47.5 miles
14	7 miles	Fartlek 2 mile w-up 4 x 1 mile Zone # 3 1/2 mile Zone #1 1 mile c-d	OFF	10 miles	OFF	6 miles	18 miles	50 miles

Week	Monday	Tuesday	Wednesday	Thursday	Friday	Saturday	Sunday	Mileage
15	7 miles	Fartlek 2 mile w-up 6 x 3/4 mile Zone #3 1/4 mile Zone #1 1 mile c-d	OFF	10 miles	OFF	Fartlek 2 mile w-up 6 x 1/2 mile Zone #3 1/4 mile Zone #1 1 mile c-d	20 miles	52 miles
16 Rec. Week	OFF	5 miles	OFF	5 miles	OFF	5 miles	10 miles	25 miles

Month Five - Intermediate Marathon Training

The fifth month is similar in structure to the 4th month, however, given the strength you've built during month four, you should be able to notch down your pace a little bit. Five to ten seconds per mile could take more than four minutes off your marathon time. Experiment this month by increasing you pace slightly and see how your body responds. You should have a good gauge on your 20 mile pace from the previous month's workout. Did you finish stronger or slower? Adapt accordingly and fine tune the engine for your race. **Avoid the temptation to walk farther than 20 miles. Walking over 20 miles takes longer to recover from and adds a risk of injury.**

Week	Monday	Tuesday	Wednesday	Thursday	Friday	Saturday	Sunday	Mileage
17	7 miles	Fartlek 2 mile w-up 2 x 1 1/2 mile Zone # 3 1/2 mile Zone #1 1 mile c-d	OFF	10 miles	OFF	Fartlek 2 mile w-up 6 x 1/2 mile Zone # 3 1/4 mile Zone #1 1 mile c-d	16 miles	47.5 miles
18	7 miles	Fartlek 2 mile w-up 4 x 1 mile Zone # 3 1/2 mile Zone #1 1 mile c-d	OFF	10 miles	OFF	6 miles	18 miles	50 miles
19	7 miles	Fartlek 2 mile w-up 6 x 3/4 mile Zone #3 1/4 mile Zone #1 1 mile c-d	OFF	10 miles	OFF	Fartlek 2 mile w-up 6 x 1/2 mile Zone # 3 1/4 mile Zone #1 1 mile c-d	20 miles	52 miles
20 Rec. Week	OFF	5 miles	OFF	5 miles	OFF	5 miles	10 miles	25 miles

Taper - Intermediate Marathon Training

Our advise for intermediate walkers' tapering for a marathon is nearly identical to that of the beginners. The sole difference is the change in fartlek workout. Since, as an intermediate walker, you've walked your fartleks at the lower end of Zone #3, continue to do so. Remember, the work is all done. The most important aspect of your training for the last two weeks is rest. It's too late to go out and make up the mileage. You need to enter your marathon well rested and ready to walk.

Week	Monday	Tuesday	Wednesday	Thursday	Friday	Saturday	Sunday	Mileage
21	7 miles	Fartlek 2 mile w-up 6 x 1/2 mile Zone #3 1/4 mile Zone #1 1 mile c/d	OFF	5 miles	OFF	5 miles	10 miles	34.5 miles
22	5 miles	OFF	5 miles	3 miles	OFF	2 miles	Marathon Day	41 miles

Recovering from a Marathon

Once the race is over, you'll probably feel it for days. When Jeff coached Team in Training he used to call it the staggered "walk" many first-time marathoners had the day after the "marathon shuffle," because people struggled walking upright and without stumbling. If you follow our training program, and wear well broken-in shoes, you should not come down with the shuffle affliction. Sure, you'll be sore for a few days, but your training will have prepared you properly.

Although laziness may beg you to take the day off after the marathon, try to get out and pedestrian walk two miles to loosen up the body. Perform a few technique drills and a lot of stretching.

Once you start to feel better, don't go right back to hard training or worse, jump into other races. It takes a good month to recover completely from the marathon. Take the first week very easy and then walk no more than 5 to 7 miles of Zone #1 walking until you've recovered.

While there are some people who have raced a marathon every week for a year, this is not a wise plan. Since building up and walking a marathon takes so much out of you, we do not recommend walking more than two marathons a year. Spacing your marathons out by six or more months gives your body the time to rebuild and come back stronger for the next one.

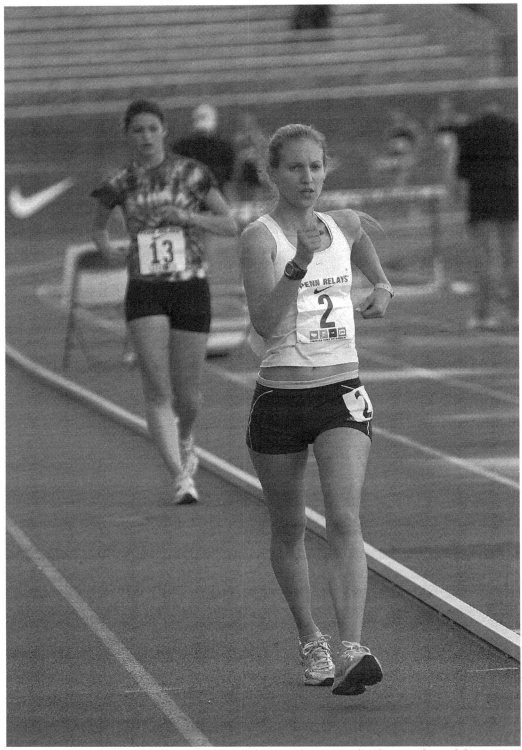

Maria Michta of Champions International, one of America's Olympic hopefuls in 2012

Chapter Ten - 50km Training

The Olympic Track and Field Program, World Championships, and World Cup offer two distances for race walkers to compete. The men compete in both the 20km and 50km events, while the women currently race at the 20km distance. The 50km is just over 31 miles long and is the longest footrace in the Olympics. It is far more grueling than running a marathon. While an Olympic medalist in a marathon is "only" running for around 2:06, the 50km is usually won in a time just under 3:40. The added time, distance and requirement to maintain technique makes participating in the 50km walk far more difficult.

To be competitive, athletes endure a high degree of stress upon their bodies, both mentally and physically. This occurs not only in the race, but also in the preparation to get to the start line. To compete, you must have both the mental and physical fortitude to withstand the pressures that are sure to come.

Mental Component of a 50km

The mental component of the 50km cannot be underestimated. Moving your legs non-stop for almost four hours for elite walkers, and five or six hours for intermediate walkers, under the watchful eye of the judges is extremely difficult. During the 50km your mind and body can play tricks on you and you must be prepared for the ups and downs that inevitably occur. The key is to focus on what helps you succeed. Technique and race day nutrition should be at the forefront of your mind. Sometimes your mind will tell you that you feel great and you should pick up the pace. Be careful, the race doesn't start until 40km. Everything else is just the warm-up. Invariably, somewhere along the way your mind will tell you that you are too tired to continue; push through it and trust your training. Be smart, be consistent, because these are the keys to a successful 50km.

In the course of my career, I have seen numerous athletes overcome obstacles both before and during the 50km. From the torrential rain and wind of the 2000 Olympic Trials to the grueling and searing summer heat of the World Championships in Osaka, Japan, the 50km can either beat you down or make you a champion.

Physical Component of a 50km

The 50km is all about training. It is about getting the miles under your legs at the right pace with the correct recovery. Almost any semi-elite athlete can walk the pace needed to excel at the 50km distance. In fact, many high school kids are already walking fast enough to walk a good 50km, but the limiting factor of the 50km isn't about speed, it is about endurance. 50km training requires large deposits into your physical bank and building the engine in order to excel. When you race a 50km, you make a much bigger withdrawal out of your bank than the shorter race walking events. In order to excel, you must make many deposits over a long period of time. The 50km isn't a distance that you just jump into. It takes years of training and preparing to be successful. For some, being successful could mean just finishing the race, while for others, it could mean winning their first and only National Championship. Either way, for those experienced athletes, the 50km could be their ticket to the Olympic Games. You must not under estimate its ability to destroy you if do not train properly.

Before you attempt to compete in the 50km, it is recommended that you have trained for the 20km for at least two to three years first and are comfortable walking 50 miles (80 km) per week. This helps ensure your body is prepared to walk the longer distances at the appropriate speed necessary for you to have a successful base for the start of your 50km training. Don't try the 50km too early in your career. In one instance, an athlete I knew competed in the 50km before he was ready. It took him 6 years to fully recover. Don't let this happen to you. Follow the TEAMS system before you attempt to move up in distance.

Hydration/Nutrition

You may think all of the hard work is done when you finish the last workout before your 50km race, but there is one additional factor that is key to your success in a 50km, proper pre- and in-race nutrition. Over the past decade I have witnessed some amazing 50km battles. The #1 factor differentiating the gold, silver and bronze medal, was one athlete's ability to stay hydrated and to get enough calories into his system.

Before the Race

You must find an electrolyte drink that does not cause problems for your stomach. You **cannot** simulate what the stomach will go through during a 50km by trying out a new sports drink on a short walk and assume, if your stomach handles the drink, it will be okay during the 50km race. You must try out any sports drink during both your longer Zone #1 sessions and during your Zone #2 sessions, because the body jostles differently with the faster paces.

Since the body cannot store enough accessible carbohydrates, you must take in simple sugars during your race. By consistently taking gels you boost your caloric balance by approximately 100 calories at a time, gaining you a huge advantages at later stages of the race. If your body can handle it, you need to take a gel every 8km to 10km during the race. Practice this as well in both your longer and harder workouts. You must get your stomach accustomed to whatever you will take during the race.

During the Race

During the race it is important you know what your body needs before it asks for it. Waiting until you are thirsty is too late. You have already passed the point at which your body needed fluid replacement. The exact amount you require is individually based. The best way to determine your fluid replacement rate it to experiment in practice. Many athletes underestimate their need. Depending upon the weather conditions, you should take in between 3 oz. to 6 oz. every 2km. In some cases, you may need even more. A lot depends on how hot and humid it is on race day. In Seville, Spain, at the 1999 IAAF World Championships, American Record holder Curt Clausen calculated exactly how much he had to drink each and every 2km to stave off his body crashing. He did this by practicing under race conditions and weighing himself before and after practice. Since

144

the primary loss of weight was due to fluid loss, he determined that he should ingest an equal amount during his race. By weighing the fluid he used as a replacement, he was able to accurately estimate how much and how often he needed to drink. There is one caveat to this method. You, too, must find out before the race how much your stomach can safely handle, depending on the conditions. It may not be feasible to take in as much as you lose.

As mentioned before, you must try to take carbohydrate rich gels every 8 to 10 kilometers. This will help you tremendously at the later stages of the race. Be aware of the caffeine level contained in many gels. Some have none, and some are loaded. Caffeine can give you a much needed boost late in the race, but it can also increase your risk of dehydration. Consult an expert before playing with significant caffeine during your race.

Developing a Schedule for 50km Race Walkers

The following is a sample schedule for an athlete training for the 50km. It assumes you've race walked for a few years and have successfully completed a 20km program two or three times before moving up in distance to the 50km. I used to say that an aspiring elite athlete had to walk at least 1:28:00 for 20km before they should venture up to the 50km distance. That is no longer the case. With the current lack of depth in the U.S., there are multiple opportunities for semi-elite athletes to excel and possibly win a National Championship. It is also an opportunity for an athlete to learn what their bodies will endure and to see what their stomach is able to handle. Still, you should never do the 50km, though, unless you are prepared for it.

Whether this is your first 50km or you are trying to improve your previous 50km performance, this schedule will help you excel. Because the schedule is Zone based, walkers of many levels can succeed with it.

The schedule starts on the first of September. We have chosen this date so you have enough time to prepare before for the annual National Championships. Since very few 50km races are held in the U.S. this seems like a reasonable target for most athletes. The schedule starts a bit earlier than the other chapters in the book, but it is imperative you begin your preparation early enough so you aren't rushing your 50km training and trying to get in shape too soon, thus missing out on the necessary mileage.

Since the 50km Nationals is typically held in the middle of February, I have chosen this as our competition date, but you may have to adjust the schedule to fit the needs of the individual season. If the date of the race changes, you must make sure that you adjust the schedule accordingly.

Phase I - Early Season Base Work for the 50km

The Early Season Base Work phase for an athlete training for the 50km lasts 8 weeks. This gives you enough time to slowly and safely build up your mileage, while also building your engine for the extreme effort that it will endure in the middle of February. The goal during this phase is to get some longer training sessions completed before adding high quality longer fartleks into the training plan.

Here is the schedule for the Early Season Base Work phase for 50km race walkers:

In week # 5 you will see that there is a lactate test. This will be a good indicator where you are at this point in the season.

Week	Monday	Tuesday	Wednesday	Thursday	Friday	Saturday	Sunday	Mileage
1	8km walk Zone #1	10km easy run	10km walk Zone #1	OFF	8km easy run	10km walk Zone #1	12km Hiking	58km Total
2	10km walk Zone #1	12km easy run	12km walk Zone #1	OFF	10km easy run	12km walk Zone #1	15km Hiking	71km Total
3	10km walk Zone #1 / 5km easy run	12km walk Zone #1	15km walk Zone #1	OFF	10km walk Zone #1 / 5km easy run	15km walk Zone #1	18km Hiking	90km Total
4	15km walk Zone #1 / 6km easy run	12km walk Zone #1	18km walk Zone #1	OFF	12km walk Zone #1 / 6km easy run	20km walk Zone #1	20km Hiking	109km Total
5	15km walk Zone #1 / 8km easy run	15km walk Zone #1	20km walk Zone #1	OFF	12km walk Zone #1 / 8km easy run	22km walk Zone #1	24km Hiking	124km Total
6	15km walk Zone #1	Lactate Test 2km w-up 7 x 2km 2km c-d / 8km easy run	25km walk Zone #1 / 30 min AJ	OFF	12km walk Zone #1 / 8km easy run	25km walk Zone #1	25km Hiking	136km Total
7	15km walk Zone #1 / 10km easy run	15km walk Zone #1	25km walk Zone #1 / 30 min AJ	15km walk Zone #1	12km walk Zone #1 / 8km easy run	30km walk Zone #1	22km Hiking	152km Total
8 Rec. week	12km walk Zone #1 / 6km easy run	12km walk Zone #1	18km walk Zone #1	OFF	12km walk Zone #1 / 6km easy run	25km walk Zone #1	12km run	103km Total

Phase II - Late Season Base Work for the 50km

The Late Season Base Work phase adds some longer fartleks into the training schedule. For those athletes coming in with a strong background in the 20km, these are going to feel slow and long. It is important, though, you follow the zones prescribed to make sure you don't peak too early and you focus on good technique. This phase lasts seven weeks.

Make sure you test your lactate on some of the longer fartlek days so you aren't pushing the workouts too fast. These should be done between 2.0 and 3.0 mmol/L, and you must make sure you are doing everything you can to recover as quickly as possible. Also, make sure you are eating and sleeping enough.

Here is the Late Season Base Work phase for 50km race walkers:

Week	Monday	Tuesday	Wednesday	Thursday	Friday	Saturday	Sunday	Mileage
9	15km walk Zone #1 10km easy run	18km walk Zone #1	25km walk Zone #1	12km walk Zone #1 8km easy run	Fartlek 3km w-up 3 x 4km/1km 2km c-d Zone # 2 6km easy run	15km walk Zone #1	30km walk Zone #1	159km Total
10	12km walk Zone #1 10km easy run	18km walk Zone #1	25km walk Zone #1 30 min AJ	12km walk Zone #1 10km easy run	Fartlek 3km w-up 3 x 5km/1km 2km c-d Zone # 2 6km easy run	15km walk Zone #1	35km walk Zone #1	155km Total
11	12km Hiking 10km easy run	18km walk Zone #1	25km walk Zone #1	OFF	Fartlek 3km w-up 3 x 6km/1km 2km c-d Zone # 2 6km easy run	12km walk Zone #1	40km walk Zone #1	148km Total
12 Rec. week	15km Hiking	12km walk Zone #1 6km easy run	18km walk Zone #1	OFF	15km walk Zone #1	15km walk Zone #1 6km easy run	25km walk Zone #1	112km Total
13	12km walk Zone #1 5km easy run	Fartlek 3km w-up 2 x 10km/1km 2km c-d Zone #2 6km easy run	25km walk Zone #1	12km walk Zone #1 8km walk Zone #1	20km Progression walk Zone #1 first 15km then Zone #2 for last 5km	15km walk Zone #1 6km easy run	35km walk Zone #1	170km Total
14	12km Hiking 8km easy run	18km walk Zone #1	Fartlek 3km w-up 4 x 5km/1km 2km c-d Zone #2 6km easy run	25km walk Zone #1	15km walk Zone #1 6km easy run	12km walk Zone #1	40km walk Zone #1	170km Total
15 Rec, week	15km Hiking	12km walk Zone #1 8km easy run	18km walk Zone #1 30 min AJ	OFF	12km walk Zone #1	20km walk Zone #1	OFF	85km Total

Phase III - In Season Racing for the 50km

The In Season Racing phase lasts for six weeks. You may be surprised that there are only two hard workouts each week, but it is extremely important to make sure you are getting enough recovery. Racing during the In Season Racing phase presents a bit of a challenge for the 50km schedule because there are typically very few races in the U.S. during this time. Over the past few years the 30km Nationals were held as early as October and as late as January. When the race is held in October it is probably too early to be of any value to your training. However, when it is held in January, it would be a great opportunity for a 30km "tempo" workout. Just be careful you don't max out your performance by walking faster than Zone #2. **Use it as rehearsal for the first 30km of your 50km instead of an all out effort.**

You may want to find a marathon which fits into your life schedule. The Las Vegas Rock and Roll Marathon is held in December and it would be a good opportunity for you to get in your longer walk in a fun and festive atmosphere. Many athletes who have trained for the 50km utilize this marathon as part of their training, but the key is to make sure you keep it at the prescribed zone. If you push too hard, it takes much longer to recover from the event than it should. Make sure these marathons stay in Zone #1 for both pace and heart rate. As you will see, this phase begins with a nice 20km walk in Zone #2. Make sure you don't push this workout past the zone prescribed because if you do, you are sure to struggle for the rest of the week, as you "carry" the tempo workout on your shoulders. You will also notice a shift from fartleks over to speedwork workouts. This gives your body a chance to recover from the hard work you have done over the previous few months. It is imperative you pinpoint exactly where and when you need to take your gels and how much fluids you need to drink in order to get in as many calories as your stomach can handle. This is the time to make sure you are using the same sports drink in the same type of "water" bottle so you become extremely comfortable using it.

Here is the In Season Racing phase for 50km race walkers:

Week	Monday	Tuesday	Wednesday	Thursday	Friday	Saturday	Sunday	Mileage
16	12km walk Zone #1 / 8km easy run	Tempo 3km w-up 20km walk Zone # 2 2km c-d / 6km easy run	25km walk Zone #1	15km walk Zone #1 / 10km easy run	12km walk Zone #1	Fartlek 3km w-up 4 x 5km/1km 2km c-d Zone #2 / #3	30km walk Zone #1	166km Total
17	12km walk Zone #1 / 6km easy run	Lactate Test 2km w-up 7 x 2km 2km c-d / 5km easy run	25km walk Zone #1 / 30 min AJ	12km walk Zone #1	Fartlek 3km w-up 2 x 10km/1km 2km c-d Zone #2 / 6km easy run	12km walk Zone #1	40km walk Zone #1	162km Total
18 Rec week	12km Hiking	12km walk Zone #1	15km walk Zone #1 / 30 min AJ	OFF	12km walk Zone #1	12km walk Zone #1 / 6km easy run	20km walk Zone #1	89km Total

Week	Monday	Tuesday	Wednesday	Thursday	Friday	Saturday	Sunday	Mileage
19	12km walk Zone #1	Speedwork 3km w-up 3 x 6km 2 min rest 2km c-d Zone #2 / 6km easy run	30km walk Zone #1 / 30 min AJ	12km walk Zone #1	Speedwork 3km w-up 5km, 4km, 3km, 2km, 1km 2 min rest Zone #2 / #3 / 6km easy run	15km walk Zone #1	35km walk Zone #1	159km Total
20	15km Hiking / 6km easy run	Tempo 3km w-up 25km walk Zone #2 2km c-d / 6km easy run	25km walk Zone #1	18km walk Zone #1	15km walk Zone #1	Speedwork 3km w-up 4 x 5km 2 min rest 2km c-d Zone #2 / #3 / 6km easy un	30km walk Zone #1	171km Total
21 Rec week	12km walk Zone #1	12km walk Zone #1	25km walk Zone #1	OFF	12km Progression walk Zone #1 first 8km then Zone # 2 last 4km	12km walk Zone #1	22km walk Zone #1	95km Total

Phase IV - Peak Season for the 50km

The Peak Season phase culminates with your 50km race. For almost five months you have thought about nothing but this race, and now the day is upon you. It is imperative you stay relaxed and you make sure you are eating and drinking enough liquids. Now is not the time to try anything new, especially your electrolyte drink. Focus on good technique and don't take any risks. If you need extra recovery time, make sure you take it. All of your hard work from the previous five months now comes to fruition.

Here is the Peak Season phase for a 50km race walker:

Week	Monday	Tuesday	Wednesday	Thursday	Friday	Saturday	Sunday	Mileage
22 Taper begins	15km walk Zone #1	Tempo 3km w-up 15km walk Zone # 2 2km c-d / 6km easy run	25km walk Zone #1	OFF	Speedwork 3km w-up 3 x 5km 2 min rest 2km c-d Zone #2/#3 / 5km easy run	12km walk Zone #1	30km walk Zone #1	133km Total

Week	Monday	Tuesday	Wednesday	Thursday	Friday	Saturday	Sunday	Mileage
23 Taper Week	15km Hiking	Speedwork 3km w-up 4 x 3km 2 min rest 2km c-d Zone # 2/#3	18km walk Zone #1 --------------- 30 min AJ or 6km easy run	15km walk Zone #1	10km walk Zone #1	3km w-up Norwegian Fartlek Zone #3 2km c-d --------------- 30 min AJ or 6km easy run	20km walk Zone #1	123km Total
24 Taper Week	12km walk Zone #1	Tempo 3km w-up 8km walk Zone # 2 2km c-d At Race Pace	15km walk Zone #1	12km walk Zone #1	10km walk Zone #1	6km walk Zone #1	50km RACE	119km Total

Recovering from the 50km

Recovering from the longest distance on the Olympic Track and Field program is a very individual affair. Typically it can take anywhere from two weeks to two months, depending on the athlete. The best lesson is to follow what Robert Korzeniowski told us many times. His advice was to make sure we were recovered before we started heavy training again so we didn't have to carry the 50km on our backs for the rest of the season. It makes sense and it follows the TEAMS philosophy. If you aren't recovered and you start to train hard again, eventually you will be withdrawing from your physical bank on every workout. Recovering from the 50km is just as important as training for it, and the quicker you recover the more you deposit into the bank.

In the days that follow, take it easy. Go for an easy run, bike ride, or aqua jog lightly. Then, after about a week, start back race walking slowly. By taking your time, you decrease your chances of an injury and you increase the chance you will be back on the road speeding along once again toward stardom.

150

Chapter 11 – Additional Training Issues

In addition to the training philosophy already dictated, there are a number of issues which relate to the multiple training schedules. Therefore, chapter 11 includes topics like acclimatization, heat related issues, and pre-race nutrition.

Acclimatization

In an ideal world, we would get up the morning of a race and step out of our backyard and the start line of the race would be right there. Sadly, this is not the reality. Big races, especially race walks, are rarely nearby. Often, these races are located far away in dramatically different climates. In order to properly prepare, one must acclimatize to the new climate. This can take anywhere from a day to up to six weeks. By acclimatizing properly, you'll be better prepared for your race.

Time Zones

If you travel across time zones for a race or are simply racing at an unusual time of day, slowly adapt your training and sleeping schedule to the time zone and race time of the competition. By adapting slowly, you do not shock your body before the race, when you need to be relaxed and getting a good night's rest. The general rule of thumb dictates you need to arrive at your race location a day earlier for every time zone you cross. However, this rule must be tempered with an athlete's individual comfort level away from home. Some athletes thrive on the change of environment, whereas, other athletes benefit from the familiar surroundings of home.

Weather

Athletes must always factor in the impact of weather upon racing. Ideally, train in or simulate the weather conditions in which you expect to race. Unfortunately, predicting weather is quite difficult. Ironically, Jeff Salvage's 20km PR was set in temperatures hovering around freezing. A scant two days earlier, the weather was in the sixties. There was no way for him to prepare on such short notice. Fortunately, 30-degree weather swings occur rarely, so a little preparation goes a long way.

If you know your race-day weather will be hot and humid, then train in hot, humid conditions. If you plan to travel to a race where conditions differ from where you live, simulate them. When Salvage trained for the Macabbiah Games, he needed to prepare to race across what amounted to be a desert. Living in Washington, DC, in July of 1989, he faced very warm and sticky conditions. Still, to prepare as best he could, he trained at noon in a sweatshirt every day.

Over the course of my career I have competed in some extreme environments. From the jungles of the Amazon river basin to the swamp lands of New Orleans, to the sweltering heat of the Spanish summer, I have had to endure some tough days in my career. Along the way, I learned some very important lessons; lessons I'm passing along to you now.

Dehydration

Staying hydrated during training and of course racing is very important. The warmer the weather the more you need to hydrate. When I was in college, hydrating was a few sips of water every six to ten miles. Thankfully when Coach Peña arrived, he instilled in us the need to drink much more than we had previously. He forced us to drink every 2km and not a few sips of water, but 6 to 8 oz. of an electrolyte drink. The old adage; "by the time you are thirsty, it's already too late," is very true. Don't wait for thirst as an indicator. Practice hydration in workouts so your stomach adapts to taking in so much fluid on a regular basis. Be aware though, you can over hydrate. Read the following section on hyponatremia.

Hyponatremia

Most athletes worry about dehydration, but there is a bigger danger to a long distance athlete, hyponatremia. As opposed to dehydration, where the body does not have enough water, hyponatremia is when it has too much water and not enough electrolytes. Often athletes flood their body with water in an attempt to stave off dehydration. This dilutes the level of sodium in the blood to dangerous levels.

The symptoms of hyponatremia range from mild to severe. They include nausea, fatigue, vomiting, weakness, sleepiness, muscle cramping, disorientation, slurred speech, and confusion. As the condition progresses, seizures or coma may occur. Hyponatremia can even lead to death. Therefore, make sure you don't just drink water, but incorporate an electrolyte drink during long and hot races as well as in long workouts.

Altitude Training

Over the course of my career I have participated in numerous altitude training camps using different training philosophies at different altitudes. It wasn't until we were researching this book that I systematically analyzed each of the training camps and their respective results. Some interesting outcomes appeared. In addition, I had the opportunity to attend the 2009 United States Olympic Committee's International Altitude Symposium in Colorado Springs in October 2009 where some of the best and brightest coaches and scientists gathered to put forth their theories on altitude training. This made me rethink the way I looked at altitude training.

While only the elite athletes will most likely be able to sacrifice the time and energy necessary to leave their homes for a month for an altitude training camp, it is important for all athletes and coaches to know the benefits of altitude training.

What is altitude training?

Altitude training is a very individual affair. Some think of it as living and training as low as 5,000 feet above sea level, while others go to the extreme of living and training at 14,000 feet. The majority of people train somewhere in between. Some subscribe to the theory of "Live High, Train Low," whereby you live at an altitude higher than where you normally train. While there are many theories about altitude training, my personal belief is that the most important aspect of altitude training, especially at the beginning of your career, is to not take too many risks. An altitude camp usually costs thousands of dollars. Don't put your investment at risk. Find someplace where you will enjoy being and where you don't feel like you are stuck in a cave without access to the internet or other fun distractions to pass the time in between your training sessions. In addition, there is a lot to be said of finding a place where the water is safe to drink. If you get sick at your training camp, you will have wasted not only your money, but an important opportunity to improve your fitness level.

At altitude the air is thinner and contains less oxygen, which makes it more difficult to breathe. The body's reaction to altitude's thinner air is the production of more red blood cells in an attempt to compensate for the lower level of oxygen. When you come back down to sea level, for a certain period of time, you will have more red blood cells than when you left. In theory this should allow you to train and race faster upon your return to sea level. Red blood cells carry oxygen, so the more red blood cells you have, the more oxygen you can carry, the more "air" you will feel your lungs have. This is very important in all events in track and field, but even more so in the race walk because of the distances competed, especially at the elite level. While the theory is simple, in practicality, it is a little more complex because if you train at altitude, your training speed will be slower due to the lack of oxygen. Therefore, a balance must be struck so you do not train too high in altitude and thus cause your body not to be prepared for faster leg turnover when you return to sea level.

Over the course of my career I trained in San Cristobal de las Casas in Chiapas, Mexico (6,000 feet), Toluca, Mexico (9,000 feet), Cuenca, Ecuador (9,000 feet), Denver, Colorado (5,000 feet) and Flagstaff, Arizona (7,000 feet). We spent anywhere from three to four weeks living and training at these locations. Since 2003, though, I have trained solely in Flagstaff. My experience there started when I had the opportunity to attend a training camp with Team Plaetzer. Training camps in Flagstaff have produced the U.S. 10km, 15km, and 20km road records as well as two Olympic Silver medals for Norway. With no risks of contaminated water or polluted air, Flagstaff elicits a peaceful tranquility that leads to improved performances

How Long Should You Stay at Altitude?

At one extreme, athletes permanently move to a high altitude setting where they live and train absorbing the benefits of a lower oxygen environment. Over the course of U.S. history, many of America's great walkers lived and trained in either Colorado Springs or the Denver area. Carl Schueler, Tim Lewis, Kevin Eastler and many others were based in Colorado. These three athletes garnered seven U.S. Olympic Team berths and many American records. For many other athletes though, living there was neither feasible nor practical, so they decided to stay at sea level and train. While it is not a requirement to train at altitude, elite athletes skipping this aspect of training are missing a great opportunity.

In my experience, the closer to four weeks you stay at your altitude training camp the better. At the 2009 USOC International Altitude Symposium, Dr. Levine advised us in his studies, he has found there was approximately a 4% gain in red blood cell count after 3 weeks of altitude training and an 8% gain after 4 weeks. While anecdotally I agreed that four weeks was superior, even I was surprised how much of a difference one extra week could make. When you first get to altitude, training is difficult. Your legs feel tired, your breathing is labored, and your heart rate is elevated. From my experience, it takes almost two weeks before you feel comfortable training at altitude.

How Quickly Will You Respond to Altitude

Everyone adapts to altitude at a different pace. Jeff Salvage has seen this first hand as he often hikes over 15,000 feet and has gone higher than 19,000 feet. Some people ignorantly feel they do not adapt to altitude, but they are really just slow responders. These people need a much longer time at altitude to adapt. In contrast, quick responders are those who acclimatize quickly and are able to start training close to their sea level paces within a short period of time. It is important for you to determine early in your career whether you are a slow or quick responder. Knowing your rate of response enables you to better plan an altitude training camp.

Keys for Training at Altitude

There are many keys to altitude training, but the biggest one I learned over the course of my career, and more specifically from my Team Plaetzer teammates, was to be careful to walk "slow" initially. Many people go to altitude and immediately feel that since they are spending money and are solely focusing on training that they have to make the most out of every session. Unfortunately that is not the case. Instead, you must allow your body to adapt to the stress of altitude before you add additional stress from training. Spend the first four to five days upon arrival only doing Zone #1 workouts. Once you begin to adapt to the lack of oxygen, the next key is as always to be consistent in your training.

A key indicator of your adaption is your heart rate, listen to it! Utilizing pace as a way to determine how fast to go will not work as pace will always be slower at high altitudes. Similarly, utilizing effort is also not going to be beneficial because the thin air is going to make every day feel difficult. The smartest way to train is by watching your heart rate. The slightest hill makes the heart rate jump quicker than you can ever imagine as the body is begging for oxygen to help power your muscles. A heart rate monitor enables you to walk in the correct zone, and therefore, get the most out of each and every session.

Coming Down from Altitude

Coming down from altitude can be a risky affair for many athletes. There will be good days and there will be bad days. The trick is to synchronize your competitions and harder training days with the days you feel better. At the USOC International Altitude Symposium this topic was touched on by almost every speaker. Their statements agreed with my anecdotal observations. It is best to compete or workout hard on the second, third or fourth days down from altitude or sometime between the 10th to the 14th day. Any sort of high intensity effort should be avoided for days five through nine. Instead, walk Zone # 1 workouts on those days. Be aware, there are days you will feel sluggish. This is normal. Your legs will feel fresh again, just be patient.

Staying Healthy

While its always important to stay healthy, it is especially so when attending an altitude training camp. During the 2009 International Altitude Symposium almost every coach and scientist who spoke noted those athletes who got sick during their time at altitude had little to no benefit from their time there. It is very important you stay away from people who are sick and you make sure your body gets enough rest and recovery. Even staying healthy, you will feel much more tired at altitude with the same amount of volume and intensity of training.

Altitude Effect vs. Training Camp Effect

One of the biggest factors which really goes under emphasized is the fact that when you are at an altitude training camp, you have, for the most part, separated yourself from the rigors of your everyday life. When solely focusing on training, whether at altitude or not, it is sure to have a positive effect on your fitness level. No more rushing off to work or even to school. Instead, while you are at altitude, you train like a full-time athlete. That gives you the best chance for success.

Iron Supplementation

Altitude camp is all about red blood cells. One of the main components of red blood cells is hemoglobin, which carries oxygen to your muscles. Without an adequate supply of iron, the body can't produce enough hemoglobin and the body will therefore have less oxygen carrying capacity. While this is a very simplified explanation of what is happening in the body, the bottom line is that if you have low levels of hemoglobin, and you go to altitude, you would be better off spending your time at sea level increasing your iron levels.

While you can take supplements, be very careful. Supplements are not FDA regulated and many things can be "thrown" into the pot while the vitamins are being made without anyone looking over the companies shoulders and verifying what is actually in there. By obtaining pharmaceutical grade iron supplements, you can greatly reduce the risk. Still, you must be careful not to take too much. Side effects include diarrhea, abdominal cramping, and in some constipation. Sitting on the side of the road crunched over because your stomach hurts is not a great way to spend your workouts

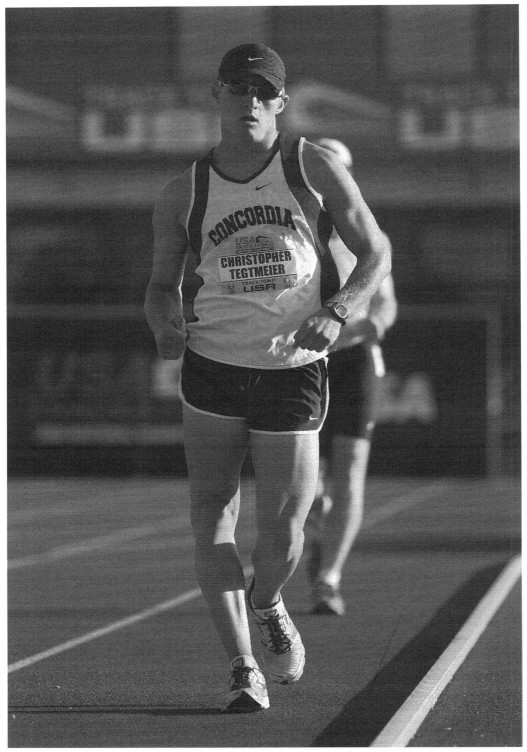

Chris Tegtmeier, one of the bright spots in American Collegiate Race Walking

Chapter 12: From Spangle Drive to the Olympic Games

Becoming an Olympian takes years of dedication, disappointments, and successes. It's rarely, if ever, a straight path to success. My story is no different.

When people hear I am a race walker, they wonder how I got involved in a relatively unknown sport. Those involved in track and field assume I was first exposed to it at the Junior Olympics, others guess I saw it on TV. However, I was fortunate enough to grow up in New York back when race walking was a part of the high school track and field program. At North Babylon Sr. High School, like most high schools in New York, the 1-mile race walk was contested just like the 1-mile run.

I started my high school track career as a respectable runner. As a freshman I ran a 5:07 for the mile and as I entered by sophomore year I was expecting to continue improving my running times. Instead, my high school coach, Coach Frank Manhardt, needed some extra points for the team, so he asked me to try race walking, which forever changed my life. While I was the best miler on the team, I was unable to score points due to a calf injury. I really didn't want to do this "funny" looking thing, but being a team player on May 14, 1988, I entered my first race walk competition. It was my 16th birthday and my gift was a 9:15 mile. Although I didn't appreciate it at time, it was one of the best birthday presents ever.

My gift, like many others, was put away shortly thereafter as I refocused my attention to soccer for the summer. Next year, when indoor track season began, I unpacked my gift and PR'd in my first race. Placing 6th in a time of 8:47 for the mile, my knees hurt so much I promised myself that I wouldn't race walk anymore. Fortunately Coach had other plans. Twelve days later I walked 8:42 and placed third, but was disqualified for the first time in my life. I was so upset and frustrated with this "stupid sport!"

I regrouped and ten days later I competed in another race. Frustratingly, I was disqualified again. I wrote in my training log, "I hate this!" Being from the old school Coach Manhardt gave me some great advice, he said, "go back out there and do the same thing again. Your technique is fine." I did exactly as he said and I was only disqualified one more time for the rest of my high school career.

I began to have more success. A few weeks later we had the league championships and I placed 2nd in a time of 8:27. This was followed by a series of races where I continually PR'd, culminating with breaking the 8-minute barrier with a time of 7:59 at the Eastern States Indoor Meet at Princeton University. After taking a few weeks off in between seasons, outdoor track started slowly. My first race was an 8:42-mile walk, however, I also ran a 5:27-mile and leaped a 31' 10" triple jump. Good fortune soon followed as I got back on track and by late in the season I broke the 7-minute barrier at the County Relays competition.

The final race of my outdoor season was the County Championships. I placed third behind Mark Barber and Paul Tavares in a time of 6:56. It was the first time that I made "All County" but I would not walk again for another five months. It was time to play soccer once again. That summer I went to Europe with a Youth National Soccer Team, so race walking was the furthest thing from my mind.

Everyone tells you your senior year of high school is supposed to be the best time of your life. For a fact I can tell you that is not the truth. For those high school athletes out there who think that it is now or never for them to succeed, I hope they continue reading my story.

Winter track of my senior year began with my first indoor race almost a minute slower than I had finished the outdoor season. A few weeks after that, one of my best friends and most talented soccer players I ever saw play the game, Tarrant Abernathy, died in his sleep. His heart just stopped. No true cause was ever found. At this point in my life, it was the most upsetting event that had ever happened to me. Tarrant was the only guy on the soccer team who had more endurance than me. I kept asking myself how this could happen? He never took drugs, he was an honest hard working athlete, and his untimely death hurt me greatly.

In high school there is no time to rest and recover. The schedule continued a few days later but the effects of Tarrant's death didn't go away. I was disqualified in my first race and I continued to race poorly. I was finally able to shake things from my head by the time the Conference Championships rolled around. I placed 2nd in a new school record time of 6:56. In the next race, the County Championships, I walked a new school record of 6:48. Sadly, I could have walked much faster. I had yet to learn the discipline of walking even splits. My 400m splits were 1:30, 1:47, 1:44 and I finished up with a 1:47. As a coach, if my athlete did this, I would go crazy.

The final indoor race of my high school career was the National Scholastic Indoor Championships in Syracuse, NY. I was very nervous before the race; it was the first time my dad was going to watch me compete. I ended up placing 4th in a time of 6:47, a new school record. Paul Tavares, who had broken the national high school record a few weeks earlier with his time of 6:11 at the Millrose Games, placed first. Ironically, Jeff Salvage paced Tavares to his record breaking time and in the process injured his knee, thus ending a promising race walking career.

As the outdoor season began, I found out my mentor, Coach Manhardt, was no longer going to be my coach. Since he was a retired teacher, he was prohibited from holding the position of head coach if a current teacher wanted the position. Instead I was going to have two new coaches whom I had never met before. Thankfully, Assistant Coach Jim DiSalvo allowed me to work with both him and Coach Manhardt. If they hadn't worked together, I would not have continued competing.

To succeed in race walking beyond high school, one has to race in distances greater than a mile. So, Coach Manhardt asked me to walk three miles straight. My first attempt was a failure. I had to break it up into three one mile repeats. Can you believe that I was able to walk under 7:00 for the mile and I had never walked 3 miles without stopping? However, eleven days later I was finally able to get the courage to try again and I walked 27:35. Pretty good for my first 5km walk. Five days later, Coach Manhardt had me step it up again. This time the goal was a 10km with a goal of walking it in 55 minutes so that I would qualify for the infamous Penn Relays. I had no idea what to expect.

Although I started out quick, each mile split was slower than the previous. I was able to luckily hang on and walk 53:23 to qualify for Penn Relays.

Ten days later, the 7 am start came bright and early that cool, clear perfect Saturday morning. There were hundreds of people in the stands, and many competitors on the start line. I split the first 5km in the same time as my time trial 10 days earlier, 25:15, but this time I stayed strong the second half. I was the top high school finisher! I lapped all of the other high school kids and finished in 7th place overall with a time of 51:12.

While I continued to improve my mile time the rest of the season, I was unable to best the speedy Tavares and placed third once again at the County Championships for the third straight time. My focus finally turned to the U.S. Junior National Championships in Fresno, California. It was the first time my dad and I had traveled by plane together, and I was really excited. I had never competed in the Junior Nationals and, in fact, I only heard of them a few weeks before the race. It was 90 degrees at the start of the race and toeing the line with me were the likes of future Olympians Andrew Hermann and Philip Dunn. The race started according to plan. I sat in the middle of the pack and planned to stay there as long as I could. Coach Manhardt's goal for me was to keep my sights on 5th place and try and stay with them as long as possible. Since this was only my second 10km, I didn't really know how to compete at a race of this distance. I saw the lap counter going down from 25, 24, 23. When it hit 10 laps to go I got excited and I pushed the pace. Shortly after, like most of us, I started to second guess. However, as Coach Manhardt taught me, once you make your move keep pushing until the end. I walked the rest of the way by myself and kept going to win my first Junior National Championship title. I couldn't believe it. Going into the race, I was the 8th fastest and now, instead worrying about that, I won the race in a 49:36.

Winning the U.S. Junior Nationals qualifies you for additional races where you represent the United States Junior National Track and Field Team. That year qualified me for two races. I thought the first time I proudly wore the U.S. National Team uniform while competing in a dual meet with Great Britain would be a success. I was wrong. Instead, it was a disaster. Starting at 11:45 am, the temperature was about 95 degrees at the start of the race in Tallahassee, Florida. Racing in that kind of heat one really needs support. Sadly there was none. The coaches called a team meeting at the same time as my race, so none of my new teammates were there to cheer for me. Thankfully, I did have Coach Manhardt and my grandfather there to lift my spirits. It was the only race my grandfather ever saw before his untimely death two years later, and the last time that I ever saw him alive. To make matters worse, there were even fewer competitors than spectators. I was the sole walker lining up to race. It sucked! I placed "first" in the 5km with a time of about 23:30 and was very disappointed with the experience. Fortunately, the second competition was in a dual meet against Canada producing better results. Although I didn't win, I finished 3rd out of 4 competitors with a time of 22:40.

Parkside Era Begins

Moving 1,000 miles away from home to Kenosha, Wisconsin, to the University of Wisconsin-Parkside was a big adjustment to me for many reasons. For the first time I had teammates who were race walkers and Coach Mike DeWitt, an expert in race walking. I will never forget showing up for the first Sunday practice and going out to train on the streets of Kenosha with over 20 other people, including my arch nemesis from high school, Paul Tavares. It was an amazing year for me. Within the first few weeks, I set TWO U.S. Junior Records in the same race. I broke the U.S. Junior 5km time with my split of 22:27 and I finished up with a new American Junior 10km time of 44:25. What an amazing day that was for me. I felt like I was on top of the world.

The feeling didn't last long. The following week I completed my first 20km in training and I abruptly crashed to earth. It took two hours and four minutes, and my legs felt like they wanted to fall off. For the next few months I had to run cross country with the rest of the walkers to maintain our scholarships.

By December we were allowed to race walk again and after a series of racing and time trials the first major challenge of the season was the Millrose Games. The legend of the Games were intimidating, but I focused on my goal and achieved another milestone in one-mile race walking: the six-minute barrier. It was a goal I never thought I would reach. I placed fourth with a time of 5:57.59, just missing winning the prize of a prestigious watch.

I didn't think I could be more nervous than at the Millrose Games, but three weeks later when I stepped on the track as the youngest walker in the U.S. Indoor National Championships, I reached a new level of anxiety. Fortunately, I got it together and walked a smart race around the 11-lap to a mile track of Madison Square Garden. I walked near dead even splits, placing second in 20:24 and qualified for my first U.S. Senior National Team trip, a dual meet with Great Britain.

Moving outdoors, I continued my progress when I returned to the Penn Relays. Older and wiser, I walked negative splits (21:50 and 21:13), breaking the 10km U.S. Junior Track record with a time of 43:03.37. While the Relays are prestigious, what mattered to the team was our big collegiate championships, the NAIA Nationals. That year they were in Stephenville, Texas, under an oppressive 85-degree heat at the start. Parkside had dominated, winning for the past eight years, so the pressure to carry on the tradition was immense for my teammates and I. While it wasn't expected of me to lead the charge, I fully expected to be in the hunt, and if the opportunity arose, try to win it for my team. The heat effected others more than myself, and before I knew it I had won my first NAIA National Championship in a time of 44:14. Back at school, in the lobby where we stretched and waited for Coach DeWitt to come down from his office before practice, there were over a hundred plaques on the walls of the National Champions, and All-Americans. I couldn't believe I would actually have my face up there with all of those legends who came before me.

There was no time for me to rest on my laurels. Four weeks later I had to defend my Junior National Championship title. It wasn't my prettiest or fastest race, but a win is a win. I walked a 44:45 with one red card and five cautions. With the racing season in high gear, over the next few weeks I had three races for the U.S. Jr. National Team. The first was a 5km race in Florida in a Junior Dual meet with Great Britain where I walked 21:13, setting a new U.S. Junior record by a mere second. The next was a 3km race and I walked 11:55 and set another U.S. Outdoor Junior record. The final race of the summer was the Pan-American Junior Track and Field Championships in Kingston, Jamaica, where I hoped to capitalize on my hot streak. The race didn't go as well as I had hoped. Due to tough competition and a less than stellar performance from myself, I placed fifth in a time of 45:23.

Ironically, Jefferson Perez, who would later become my race walking hero, placed second in the race. In just five more years he would change the race walking world forever by winning Ecuador's first ever Olympic Gold Medal in Atlanta in 1996.

Having one of the most successful freshman years in U.S. race walking history, I looked forward to building upon it. Sadly, fate had another plan. As my sophomore year began, I started to have some pain behind my left knee. After limping around for weeks I entered my one and only race of the season. It was the last time that I would walk for months, and my last race for the next year and a half.

I was still struggling at the beginning of my junior year. The pain in my left knee continued to hamper my ability to race walk. Instead, I ran cross country with the girl's team. By the middle of September I finally got an MRI and a bone scan. The results were not encouraging. I had a stress fracture in the back of my knee and bursitis. The doctor and Coach DeWitt decided I would run three days a week, which enabled me to recover while still keeping in touch with the team.

Four weeks later I started to race walk again, albeit slowly. By January, I started to train a bit more and I entered my first time trial in 18 months. A 3km indoor race at UW-Platteville in which Al Heppner and I were the only competitors. Freshman Heppner sat on me the whole race and then sprinted by the last few hundred meters. Frustrating as it was to have someone *float* by me due to the lack of judges, I still had to be happy walking a 13:06 after so much time off. Coach, the team, and I all kidded Heppner over the years for his *Platteville* technique.

Training at an elite level is always a challenge during the winter in Kenosha. Weeks on end of sub zero temperature, combined with massive snowfall due to the Lake Michigan effect, sent us crawling down into the basements of the college buildings. That winter was an extremely tough one, even for Kenosha. We had to train a lot in the basement on the hard cement floor. This did not help my recovery much. The slow progress led to frustration between Coach Dewitt and myself. Compounding this, we rolled into spring with a relentless schedule of time trials and races.

The first significant challenge since getting injured was to regain my title as NAIA Champion. Not having prepared as I wish I could have, I hoped I had enough muscle memory to pull out my 2nd championship. The race materialized into a battle with my roommate Rob Cole. With a mile to go, I tried to pass Rob, but his wandering elbow deterred my progress. I attempted again with three laps to go, but Cole had some of the sharpest elbows on the race walking scene. With two laps to go I took off and won my second NAIA Championship title in a time of 20:50. It felt awesome to win again after all of the struggles that I had to overcome. My ever supportive dad once again was there to cheer me on, providing the positive reinforcement I needed.

As was the norm, I flew home once school ended. Doug Fournier, who was one of the best walkers in the country and a Parkside graduate, lived on Long Island, so we would frequently train together.

A few weeks later, we headed to Eugene, Oregon, the home of Steve Prefontaine, to compete in my first USATF 20km Outdoor Nationals. My Dad, Doug and I flew to Oregon together. The race was at 3pm in the afternoon and the temperature was 85 degrees. I started off a bit faster than coach's plan, going through 5km in 22:44. After that I started to struggle. Doug started out slower and moved up through the pack and finished in an amazing 3rd place. I just got slower and slower. I finished in 1:34:49 and placed 10th. I was disappointed because I had hoped to make the World University Games team, but instead I qualified for the now defunct Olympic Festival.

The Olympic Festival was held in San Antonio, Texas, on the first of August. They clearly didn't pick the location with distance athletes in mind. To say it was hot would be an understatement. However, with solid training under my belt since Nationals, I was ready to give the 20km another try and had learned my lesson about pacing. Gary Morgan, Curt Clausen, Curtis Fisher and Don DeNoon were walking about 20 meters ahead of Jonathan Matthews and I. Jonathan kept yelling at them because he said the real race started after 10km. I knew what it felt like to go out too fast and crash and I tried my best to be as careful as possible. By 10km Jonathan was proved correct and we surged past them. He took off from me after that, but without his help, I wouldn't have been able to get the Silver medal and finish in 1:33:27.

My senior year started with a change. Instead of running, we were allowed to race walk in the fall. At first this sounded like a blessing, but the longer season coupled with endless time trials took its toll. In better shape earlier than usual, I flew to Detroit to compete in the Alongi meet, but this time I wouldn't be competing in the Junior 10km event; instead it would be the Senior 20km race. I was in pretty good shape, and my first 5km was 21:55, my second 22:03 for a 10km split of 43:58. I felt strong and ready to break the 1:30:00 barrier, but I was walking with Gary Morgan, the hometown favorite, and I started to pick up DQ calls. At 16km I slowed down but at 18,975 meters the head judge flashed the red paddle in my face and told me to stop. It was the first time I had been disqualified since my senior year in high school. Will Van Axen, in the Junior 10km, broke my 10km Junior American record in 43:18.

The following weekend I flew to compete in the USATF 5km Nationals and crossed the line in second place, but once again I was disqualified. I couldn't believe it. I questioned what I was doing wrong, but had no answers. Since we focused on training as opposed to technique, I had no clue what I should do to correct it. The only advise I could follow was my high school coach's advice, just to go out there and do the same thing.

As the new year began, once again we started with the many races and time trials. The first significant race was the Millrose Games where I finally PR'd again. Walking a 5:57.35, it was my first PR in any distance since I was a freshman almost 4 years earlier. Following my success, we continued with the intense schedule of time trials then flew to Atlanta to compete in the U.S. Indoor Nationals. Again I crossed the finish line only to be disqualified for the third time out of the last four races that were not in Wisconsin.

As the outdoor season began, I started to walk longer and longer on Sundays but almost every Saturday was a time trial or race. In April we had a special Intermediate National Team trip for those between 20 to 23 years of age. The 20km race they chose was at 6,000 feet in Pueblo, Mexico. This was one of the most memorable races of my life because Philip Dunn, Andrew Hermann, Al Heppner and I were competing on the same team for the very first time. I remember walking with

Al through 15km. We had just passed Andrew and Philip and were walking pretty strong. I looked over at Al when we were about to go up the hill on the course and I said, "Al, just please help me up the hill. Please stay with me." Al looked at me, smelt blood, and being the competitor he was dropped a gear and me in an instant, and gained a PR!

After about four more time trials we had our NAIA Outdoor Championships once again, this time at Azusa Pacific in California. I won the 5,000m for the third time in a new meet record time of 20:47. We finished up the season at the U.S. Outdoor Nationals in Knoxville, TN, on June 18th, 1994. The 20km start was 8am. I ended up placing 7th in a time of 1:31:18. It was my PR, and the top 10 in the race all finished in under 1:32:04.

Normally people graduate college after four years and although I had enough credits to do so, I decided to stay at school for what we called the "super senior" year. Since I had a year of eligibility left, I really wanted to become the first 4-time NAIA Champion in the history of the school. It would be a very interesting year to say the least.

During the summer months I had the ability to work a lot, 50-60 hours a week, and I took advantage of it. I was training as best as I could. When the summer ended and I had to hand in my training log to Coach DeWitt, he ripped into me. He wrote in my training log, "Do you think 14 days off (25%) is good? I think it stinks. If you get hurt, or miss making the Olympic Trials or even the Olympic Team think about your 75% summer dedication. It's rotten!" I was stunned. His note made such a huge impression on me I still have it attached to that training log. While he was right, the scholarship I had didn't pay for housing or food, so I had no practical choice. I moved into an apartment with Al Heppner to cut costs, and Al became like a brother to me. During that semester, I joined the guys cross country team for the first time. It felt great to be part of the guys team. The catch was we had to race walk every Sunday with Coach DeWitt. Our first Sunday back we did 12 miles. For the next 4 weeks we walked 15 miles. We continued to add distance, culminating on Christmas eve when Will Van Axen, Dave Michelli and I had the longest walk of our lives, one I will never forget. We walked 30 miles. This was part of Coach's 50km training without doing the 50km. The goal was to make us stronger. A few days later, Will, Dave and myself did 3 x 4 miles with 5 minutes rest. It was 30 degrees, but something started to happen to me again, behind my left knee was beginning to get a little sore. I was again forced to take more time off.

While I was struggling, my teammate Will Van Axen placed 6th at the World Cup Team Trials with a big PR time of 1:29:40. It was a glorious day for us because Will was the first one of us to qualify for the Olympic Trials the next year. That week we had a team meeting, one I will never forget. Coach DeWitt could tell we were all very excited about Will qualifying for the Olympic Trials and the possibilities of some of us qualifying later in the year. Some of the athletes even talked about the possibility of maybe even making the Olympic Team. We had no clue what the time standards were; we just knew once we qualified there was a chance. DeWitt wasn't very happy with this and he told us we should get those thoughts out of our heads now and that none of us would make the Olympic Team in 1996 in Atlanta. Will and I were crushed.

I still couldn't walk, but I could run, so for the next few weeks I ran Will's workouts with him to try and help him along. I saw another doctor and he said I should get orthotics to correct a leg length discrepancy. I was willing to try anything to get better and get back walking again to help my team. By the end of March I was able to walk most of the training again, although I was slower. It was great to be back. I started to feel a lot of pressure to hurry up and get in shape because of the NAIA meet was in just two months. I did the best I could every training session. I lifted weights, did abdominal work, anything I could to be healthy. By the end of April I walked a 10km at Parkside in 45 minutes. The following weekend flew to Philadelphia for the Penn Relays. I walked my "post Junior PR" in 43:47, placing 5th.

After graduation I competed in my last NAIA Outdoor Championships. There was a non-Parkside athlete named Chad Eder who had a lot of talent and we were worried about Parkside losing our streak of consecutive wins. Will Van Axen was a team player who wasn't personally concerned about winning the race. He wanted to see me win my forth NAIA Championship. Something the *ghosts* of Parkside had never done. The ghosts were those who came before us: Heiring, Kaestner, and Stauch. We had heard stories for five years about how great these guys were, but not once did they ever come out and talk to us and help us. As a young impressionable athlete, it was very hard to train there with the ghosts always looking over my shoulder telling me that I didn't do this work out as fast as they did, or that I didn't race as fast as they did. It was now my turn to do something that they couldn't do.

Will decided there was one way to beat Chad and that was to take it out hard and make him suffer from the beginning. I agreed. Will took out the pace in 3:58 for the first kilometer. In the 85-degree temperature, we went through the next kilometer in 4:03, and Will had just dropped off the pace. Chad took the lead, with me behind him and Al behind me. The next km was 4:10. I decided to start playing games with him. I would get up beside him and test him. I did this three times just like Coach Manhardt had taught me in high school. I had to dig deep but I kept thinking about Coach Manhardt and all of the miles he had ridden his bike with me over the years. I thought how proud he would be of me if I succeeded. When we hit four laps to go, with my dad in the stands, I made a huge move and did not look back. I won my fourth NAIA Nationals in a new meet record time of 20:39. Will taught me a lot about teamwork that day as his grin was as big as mine.

On the flight back to Wisconsin, I went up and sat next to Coach DeWitt. I told him I had made a decision and that I was going to go down to La Grange and train with Bohdan Bulakowski. It was one of the hardest decisions I had ever made. At Parkside you are basically taught that it can't be done outside of Kenosha. I wanted a chance to be an Olympian and I knew the cold weather of Wisconsin would just get me injured. The decision was so difficult that I cried. Coach Dewitt gave me an amazing opportunity. I had a scholarship at the most famous *race walking* college in U.S. history. I questioned if I was being disrespectful to him by leaving. Switching coaches like this was a very difficult decision. I stayed up many a nights tossing and turning thinking about it. But after that race at NAIA's I knew I had potential. I gave myself a two percent chance of making the Olympic Team the next year. Coach had given me a 0% chance a few months before. I decided to roll the dice.

My final race as a Parkside athlete occurred on June 18th, 1995. It was the USATF Outdoor National Championships 20km in Sacramento, CA. Everyone was there. Allen James took the lead from the beginning and he never looked back. He finished up in an amazing time of 1:24:46. Meanwhile, I had started off in a nice pack going through 5km in 21:55. I then went through 10km in 44:04. I was pretty happy with how things were going so far, but after 10km I started to slow once again. I fought hard and I ended up placing 6th in a time of 1:29:20. The ironic thing was that as I turned the last corner with 100m to go, I was in 5th place and out of nowhere, Curt Clausen came storming past to beat me by .02 of a second. He had thought he had to beat me in order to go to the World University Games in Fukouka, Japan, that summer, but in fact both of us had qualified.

Soon after I began getting my workouts from Bohdan. The mileage increased, but the pace was slower. As the weeks progressed, I became stronger and more confident. I began to feel like a professional athlete. My first race under Bohdan was the World University Games in Japan. Curt and I were there together and a brotherly bond began to grow between us. The race started off fantastic. I went through the first 10km in 43:50, but soon the 80+ degree temperatures got to me and I crashed really hard. I averaged 4:23/km the first 10km and 5:12/km the last 10km, finishing up in 1:35:36. After 12km I just gave up mentally, I would use this race as a motivator for the next few months.

My next race didn't go very well either. I did the U.S. National 5km Championship. I ended up with a 21:18, but it was for nothing because I was disqualified. The following weekend I redeemed myself, placing second in the Atlantic City boardwalk race. It was the first time that I won money race walking. The $250 prize money was a nice way to start the next chapter of my life, training in LaGrange, Georgia.

LaGrange Begins

When I arrived to the "I Train in LaGrange" program, I was very impressed. Allen James, Rob Cole, Mike and Michelle Rohl, Herm Nelson, Dave McGovern, and Andrew Hermann were all part of the training group. I looked forward to training with an Olympic race walker for the first time. Unfortunately, I arrived too late to take advantage of the free housing but found a small cheap apartment nearby. Bohdan's training methodology was very different than Parkside's. We started off very slow, taking almost 4 weeks of easy walking before we walked our first 20km workout. We really focused on technique, which I clearly needed. That really paid off as the first few indoor races all led to PR's and more importantly, no disqualifications.

For the next few weeks training was going ok, but the group in LaGrange was starting to disintegrate into factions. While I was used to everyone training together, here there were groups that would not train with other groups. I was willing to train with everyone, attempting to be a middle man trying to bring everyone together.

One of the great side benefits of race walking is travelling and living in different locations. On March 8th many of us traveled to San Cristobal de las Casas in Chiapas, Mexico, for our first altitude training camp. Andrew Hermann's parents had a small place there, so we could train without having to pay for housing. With no work, no English TV and virtually nothing to do but concentrate on the task at hand, training was amazing. I smashed my highest weekly training total of 127kms by averaging 155km/week for the 4 weeks. There were no 7-11 stores to pick up a Gatorade, we walked with only a few pesos in our pockets to buy cold cokes in plastic bags with straws sticking out.

I returned home and flew to Budapest, Hungary, to meet up with Dave McGovern and Mark Versano for a 20km race. Dave and I decided to walk together and we went through 10km in 42:22. We couldn't believe it. It felt easy and we were able to talk the whole time. By 16km though, Dave's notorious stomach acted up and he started viciously throwing up. I stopped and yelled at Dave that we had come this far, I wasn't going to finish this race without him. Dave got back up and started walking again. With only 3km to go, we were moving fast once again. Our next two kilometer splits were 4:15 and 4:12, with my last split at 4:08. I walked a PR by almost five minutes. McGovern, inconceivable as it was, finished ahead of me. It was the first time I had negative splits in a 20km race, and my time of 1:24:35 made me the fourth fastest American ever. Dave walked 1:24:29.

Next, I traveled back to America to work as Andrew Hermann's pit crew at the 50km Olympic Trials. Andrew raced great, placing 2nd, but didn't have the time standard for the Olympics so he would have to try and do another 50km later in the year. Two weeks later we all flew to Europe to compete in two Grand Prix races. The race was going to be on the track and I felt ready for it. Having lost to Allen James in all three indoor races, as he so *graciously* reminded me, was something I was determined not to repeat. Allen and I walked the first 3km together, but by 4km I had two red cards on the board. Even though the pace was easy, I slowed down to focus on technique. At 10km the Moreno brothers from Colombia lapped me and I hitched a ride. We caught Allen at 15km and as soon as I passed him, he *graciously* dropped out. Finishing in 1:25:28, I placed 5th overall and achieved my 20km track PR.

A week later we traveled to Eisenhuttenstadt, Germany, to particpate in the largest race walk I had ever competed. With 85 walkers on the start line, I was in awe of the number of walkers trying to achieve Olympic time standards. At that time the "A" standard was 1:24:00. If two Americans walked under that barrier, they would virtually lock in their spots on the 1996 Olympic Team. Reaching that goal would get the ghosts from Parkside off my shoulder forever. The race started off and I got *dragged* along to a 5km split of 20:33. Slowing slightly for the next 5km, I went through 10km in a PR of 41:30. I was shocked. I never expected to be on such a fast pace. Clocking a 21:12 for the next 5km, I began to struggle. To achieve the "A" standard it meant I couldn't slow by more than 6 seconds for the final 5km. Sadly, by 18km I was really hurting and the "A" standard slipped away. Still a PR is always an achievement and I dug deep to walk faster than any American other than Tim Lewis. My last kilometer I walked a 4:08 to finish up in 1:24:14, more than five minutes faster than I had walked at Parkside.

After the race I had a long talk with Bohdan and he decided to send me back up to altitude, this time I was going to go to Colorado Springs and train with Andrzej Chelinski, which was a lot of fun. The training camp went very well and I knew leaving there I would be ready to fight at the Olympic Trials. There were five of us in the U.S. with a "B" standard, so only one of us would be able to go. It was winner take all. The race started in the Atlanta Olympic Stadium, with myself and Allen James leading a pack of five walkers. Behind us was another pack of about five athletes. By 5km, Philip Dunn, Curt Clausen, and Gary Morgan had joined us up front walking the streets of Atlanta hoping for a spot on the Olympic Team. Most of the other guys had brushed off Gary Morgan as too old, but not me. I respected Gary tremendously because, he said to me many times, "Let me tell ya, I won the one that counted." Gary was referring to the steam bath of the 1988 Olympic Trials in Indianapolis in which he beat Tim Lewis to clinch forever his status as an Olympian. By 12km the battle was between myself and Curt. He made a move first, putting on an unmatchable surge. Staying in the hunt, I worked my way back to him by 17km. However, as we approached the last turn, Curt had another surge in him and he broke away, winning in a time of 1:29:50. I placed 2nd in a time of 1:30:27. Thirty-six-year old Gary Morgan placed third in a time of 1:31:00. I was now the alternate for the 1996 Olympic Games. That afternoon, Andrew Hermann and I met with our then race walking chairman, Bruce Douglas, and we formulated a 4-year plan to get us onto the 2000 Olympic Team. That plan was to start up a residency program at the Olympic Training Center in Chula Vista, California.

When the gun went off at the 1996 Atlanta Olympic race walk, I was there as a spectator. Instead of pouting, I viewed the Olympics as an opportunity. While Curt's race didn't go exactly according to his plan, walking 1:31:30 and placing 49th, my friend Jefferson Perez from Ecuador won his country's first Olympic Medal in the 20km in 1:20:07. To this day it was one of the most awe inspiring performances I have ever seen. Seeing a humble athlete from a poor country beat up on the wildly successful Russian machine gave me hope that one day I might accomplish equal success.

The first major post-Olympic championship was the Sallie Mae 5km Nationals in Pennsylvania and it was the battle for the short distance crown. Gary Morgan blasted out with a 3:52 first kilometer. Dave McGovern and I hung in there and by 3km Gary had to drop back with some judging issues. From then on it was Dave and I battling back and forth. With 1km to go, Dave had a 5 meter lead on me, but with 600m to go, I put on a huge surge. I came through in 19:59, winning my first U.S. Championship, and my first American Record on the Senior level.

The final race of the season was the Pan-Am Cup in Manaus, Brazil, and one where I would learn patience. Excited by my first visit to South America, I made a huge mistake. Under oppressive heat and humidity, Allen James and I took the lead from the start. Why I did this, I still can't understand. In the end, I placed 13th in a horrible time of 1:41:41. At least I got to see the Amazon River, which passed right by the edge of the course. Its reputation for size did not disappoint as I could barely see from one side to the other.

ARCO Begins

After a few agonizingly slow months of waiting around, the paperwork for our residency program at the Olympic Training Center was complete. I moved in at the same time as Philip Dunn and Will Van Axen. Under the tutelage of Bohdan we increased our mileage dramatically. The first month we averaged over 150km per week. It was such a huge help to not have to worry about food and rent expenses.

By March 1st we had the U.S. Indoor Nationals in Atlanta and I was feeling ready to go. I figured I could walk well under 19:45, possibly around 19:30, but it was not to be. This was Allen James' last race before he retired and I really wanted to try and beat him, but I could not muster the strength to do it. I ended up finishing 2nd in 20:12, after a huge battle with Philip Dunn the last km. Allen won the race in 20:07.

We had the first 20km of the 1997 season at the World Cup Trials in Virginia. This was a very memorable race because Curt, Philip, Andrew and myself all walked together for 15km. It was then that I said to myself, "*con cojones,*" and I took off. Our first 10km was 43:24, but my next 10km was 42:41, and my last 5km under 21 minutes. I was pretty excited about this race. It was the first time in almost 9 months I had been under 1:30:00. My final time was 1:25:56.

At the end of April we traveled over to Podebrady, Czech Republic to compete in the World Cup. In the best shape of my life, I hoped for success. The first 5km was 20:40 and all looked like my plan was falling into place. Then, disaster struck. For the first time in my life I had to hit the port-a-potties. Whenever I would regroup, I had to go again. By the end, I had to make five pit stops and I was barely able to beat the barefooted race walker from Malaysia. I ended up placing 103rd, my worst performance in international competition. Dealing with my own disappointment wasn't the worst part, it was how upset Bohdan was with me. I don't think he talked to me for three days. The rest of the season didn't go very well, with me finishing in third place at the U.S. Outdoor Nationals in a time of 1:30:00. The only positive aspect of the season was the New York Athletic Club asked me to join their team.

After a few weeks off, we started training again. Curt Clausen joined us as well as Andrew Hermann, Al Heppner, Danielle Kirk, Susan Armenta and Margaret Ditchburn. Soon after Bohdan started to get upset, and rightfully so, about coaching us for free. While he was provided free housing and food, we weren't able to pay him. We decided to each pay $2,000 to Bohdan. While I knew it would be difficult, it was the only thing we could do to keep Bohdan there. Sadly, the added expense was too much for Will Van Axen. The Olympic fire inside him wasn't strong enough, so he left. The rest of us scrambled to come up with the money. Thankfully, Elaine Ward and the North American Race Walking Institute stepped in to help by raising all the money needed for Bohdan's salary.

Training was going well except for a small pain in my lower abdominal muscles. The focus was on heavy mileage again as we prepared for my first 50km race. I was excited about this new challenge and was logging 30km-40km for my long workout each week. My goal was to break 4:00 hours, and it looked attainable.

The 1998 50km Nationals were being held in Palo Alto, CA, and although I planned to walk with Curt, his pace was too fast, so I had to slow down and walk alone. Even though a torrential storm hit by 20km, the first 30km was relatively easy. They say the 50km race starts at 40km. This adage proved true. I was comfortable through 42.5km and then really started to crash. I went from walking my 10km's in under 48 minutes, to around 54 minutes for the last 10km. With 300m to go, my legs were in excruciating pain and I did not want to walk another step. The cold, wind, and rain finally got to me. Like a guardian angel, Carl Schuler, an American Olympic legend, came running down the path and told me to finish the race. With him rooting me on, I was able to push through the final 300 meters and finish my first 50km in 4:05:35. Like many 50km walkers before me, my first words were "I will never do this stupid thing again."

Three weeks later were the 1998 U.S. Indoor Nationals in Atlanta. My goal was to stay behind Curt until sometime after 3km. Our splits the first 3km were 4:03, 3:59, 4:02. I walked right behind him until about a mile to go, then I made my move. The next two kilometers were both in 3:54, and I was able to become the third American to ever break 20 minutes indoors for the 5,000m in a time of 19:54. It was my first U.S. Indoor title and only the second National Championship of my career. Still having a lot of pain in my abs, this win helped cure the pain for a little while.

Although training was going well, I suffered through a race in Bergen, Norway, as well as one in La Coruna, Spain. I was getting very discouraged. Upon our return to the States, Curt Clausen and I went straight to Chicago in May for the U.S. 15km Championships. Curt and I had another one of our epic battles. We started slow and let Mike Rohl lead the first 5km in 23:00. Our next 5km was a bit faster, 21:13. Curt and I really started to hammer each other. With two km to go we were cruising and that is when I made one big push at the end, with my last 5km in 20:32 and a finish of 1:04:36. Curt finished nine seconds back. My lower abs hurt terribly after the race. No one at the Training Center could figure out what was causing the pain. Doctors would volunteer for two weeks at a time and every one of them, over eight months, looked at me but to no avail.

During that season our team bond grew stronger and stronger. At the U.S. Outdoor Nationals in New Orleans on June 19th, 1998, the goal was for us to walk the 20km as a team and try and counteract the 96 degrees and 90% humidity. Confident as ever, Curt took the lead. Scared of the oppressive conditions, everyone reluctantly held back. I garnered enough strength and I went up and walked next to him. By 7km though, Curt started to struggle and fell back. I walked alone with just my dad and high school friend cheering me home. Entering the final tunnel into the stadium alone I couldn't believe I would win a *real* one. While the other national championships are an accomplishment, it's really the 20km and 50km that define elite success in race walking. Although many people were critical of the fact it was the slowest winning time in 25 years, it was a huge accomplishment for me. Besides the heat, I was still struggling with my abdomen pain. It was this injury that basically ended my season after a disappointing disqualification at the Goodwill Games later that summer.

By the time I was ready to walk again, many changes occurred within the team. The biggest change was one at the top. Coach Enrique Peña, the coach of Jefferson Perez, replaced Bohdan. We were reluctant to see Bohdan go, but felt the change was for the better. In addition, John McLaughlin stepped in to assist Elaine Ward with our fundraising, as Peña's salary was higher. At this point I had to focus on resolving the horrendous pain in my abdomen. Three cortisone shots directly into the pubic symphysis, the space directly between my two hip bones in the center of my body, didn't help at all. I was finally given the bizarre sounding diagnosis - osteitis pubis. I decided to have pelvic floor repair surgery and suffered through an incredibly painful recovery. It was predicted I would be race walking in four weeks, instead I was just starting to sit up straight. Walking without pain was out of the question. Progress remained slow for five months. On Christmas I gave myself a present. I race walked ten minutes.

A few weeks later, I rejoined the team. Within a few weeks, I was back racing. Amazingly, in my first race I set a 3km PR in 11:33. The PR came with a price. The following week I began to have problems once again and was treated with more shots.

Two weeks later I left for Atlanta to defend my Indoor Championship title and won primarily due to pacing myself. The next few weeks seemed like a blur as everything seemed to fall into place perfectly. With Enrique as our new coach, we had a renewed sense of motivation. Within a week of the Atlanta race, we did a 3km and 5km race at the Olympic Training Center on the track. I ended up breaking the U.S. 3km track record in 11:19 and Curt ended up breaking the U.S. 5km record in 19:35. Jefferson Perez had then joined us and everyone was excelling under the training of Enrique and mentorship of Jefferson.

My first 20km under Enrique saw me place second to Jefferson at the World Cup Trials in a time of 1:23:50. It was the first time I broke 1:24:00. A few weeks later, I became the first American to break 40 minutes for 10km, walking 39:43 at the Penn Relays. Enrique's early success gave us great confidence. He had answers for everything and if something felt off for us, he was able to adapt quickly. My first international race of the season was the IAAF 1999 World Cup in France. I was on such a high after my 10km I thought I was going to place in the top 10. I went out the first 5km with the lead pack in 20:29, then I started to struggle. I finished in 1:27:20 to place 35th.

After a few more races in Europe it was time to compete at the USATF Outdoor Nationals in Eugene, Oregon. Curt and I walked together for the first km in 4:16, but then he thought it was too slow and dropped it down to 4:02. I knew the pace was too fast for me, so I just kept walking consistence kilometers right around 4:12. By 8km I had caught Curt and we stayed there until 16km. I then made one of the biggest blunders of my career. The course was a 1km loop and for some reason, when we hit 16km, I thought it was 17km. I felt that since I was the fastest in America at the shorter distances that I would be able to make a push to the end. I started my kick. I went from 4:11 a km with Curt to 4:05 and then a 4:07. I looked up at the time clock and lap counter and I realized that I had made a huge mistake. I knew I could hold on for one more km, but two more? I didn't think so. I slowed down to 4:13/km to catch my breath from 18km to 19km. By this point, Curt had caught me and we were walking stride for stride but I was determined to fight to the end. Since Curt didn't surge at 16km like I had, he still had something left in his tank. He pushed one last time to walk his final km in 3:55 to my 4:00. I walked my fastest last km of a 20km and I got dusted doing it. The effort I put forth in that race was intense and I would not recover for the rest of the season.

We began working on the 2000 Olympic season. Since I missed the previous Olympic Team, I was determined to do it this time. On October 5th, 1999, the pain returned in my lower abs. I was more frustrated than ever. Dr. Cattey in Milwaukee performed minimally invasive surgery. Just two small incisions and five hernias were repaired. He said they were probably the problem all along. I rested two weeks, and my Olympic preparation began in earnest. I rejoined the team by Christmas.

I got in shape very quickly. On Feb 12th, the day before the 2000 50km Olympic Trials, we set up a 20km race on the track in Sacramento. This was my first real race back and I was excited. I walked 1:24:25, breaking Allen James' U.S. 20km track record by a mere 1.5 seconds, walking 43 seconds over the last 200m to do it. The next day I watched Curt, Andrew, and Philip walk their way to the 2000 Olympic Team. I also watched as Al Heppner, while having the third Olympic position locked up, succumb to hyperthermia and collapse on the sidelines. It was the beginning of Al's problems that would end suddenly on February 19th, 2004.

A few weeks later the U.S. Indoor Nationals were again held in Atlanta. Curt and I walked together for the first few kilometers, but I was finally able to break away and cross the tape in 19:32 to win my third consecutive Indoor Championship. The following week we traveled to Cuenca, Ecuador, to train with Jefferson Perez in his home town. The altitude was around 8,500 feet. It was awesome to be in the home town of my hero, to train on the same courses as he did, in a stadium that was named after him, and to suffer through the training like he did. Training did not go very well for me. Even though I averaged less than 100km per week, I struggled almost every day. I had a few good workouts but I couldn't get any consistency in my training. Jefferson was a saint. One day after training he handed me his Olympic gold medal to help inspire me. I couldn't believe I was actually holding it!

From the heights of Ecuador I was inspired but performed poorly at the Pan-Am Cup in Mexico, and several races in Europe which ended with disappointing finish times, and a disqualification. But in the process I learned a valuable lesson. The higher the altitude the less I seemed to gain from it. Almost two months after leaving Cuenca, I walked a 1:25:47 20km. While not a PR, it put me back on track.

For the next eight weeks my only goal was to make the Olympic team. I decided nothing would get in the way of joining my teammates in Sydney. Enrique was instrumental in helping me regain my focus. We once again went to three speedwork sessions per week. I did everything possible to maximize my recovery from the brutal 7 x 2km workouts and the 3 x 5km workouts.

As the Olympic Trials approached, I was extremely nervous. While there were just two of us with the Olympic "B" standard, it was still very nerve racking. Curt was injured and most people would have said it would be an easy win for me, but I did not under estimate Kevin Eastler. He was very talented and highly motivated. There was also Andrew Hermann, the 50km Olympian who had pummeled me every race upon our return from Cuenca. I knew it would be a fight and I would have to walk very fast to win the race and clinch a spot on the team. Jefferson, who had been in San Diego training with us, flew up to Sacramento to cheer us on. As I was warming up, Jefferson walked with me and said, "Congratulations." I asked him what that was for, and he said, "for making your first Olympic Team." Being a little superstitious, this made me really nervous.

Kevin and I walked together for the first 12km of the race. It was at that point Kevin received his first caution and slowed down, while I dropped the hammer, going from 4:15 pace to under 4:10/km. By 15km I had a 30 second lead and I knew that all I had to do was maintain my speed. As I entered the stadium I could hear the roar of the 15,000 fans coming to life. I had to walk just 100 more meters and with each step I took closer to the finish I wished that I could just stop and enjoy the amazing feeling of the crowd cheering for me. As a race walker we don't often experience this in America, but the Olympic Trials are a special event. I came through the line in a new Olympic Trials meet record time of 1:25:41. *I could now call myself an OLYMPIAN!!*

While preparing for the Olympics, we decided to help Kevin have one more shot at making the team. Given the complicated permutations for qualifying for the Olympics, if both Kevin and I could walk the "A" standard, we would both get to go. We set up a race on a local track and we asked Elaine Ward to organize the judges for us. Kevin, Curt, Andrew, and myself, all set a pace to help Kevin. We went through the first 5km in 20:42, but it was a bit faster than the others were able to hold, so they fell off the pace. By 12km it was clear Kevin wouldn't achieve the standard and he dropped out. I ended up walking 1:23:40 to regain the American Record that Curt had previously broken in May. The next day, we left for Sydney.

My First Olympic Games

It took almost 20 hours to get to from Los Angeles to Sidney, and then on to Brisbane where we would train prior to the Games. We immediately went back to our training routine. We had a hard workout every other day for the next three weeks. This included two fast 20kms; one at 1:29:42 and the other at 1:25:55, the fastest 20km I'd had in training. I truly thought I had a shot at a medal. Two days later I did 10 x 1km in the Olympic Village, 500m out and 500m back. After the third or fourth interval I started to have a pain in my piriformis, near the upper part of my hamstring. Coach wasn't there because he went to help Jefferson with his workout. Instead of being smart and stopping, I didn't want to be a wimp and quit, so I kept going. That night at the Opening Ceremonies it was really flaring up, but the pride of walking into the Olympic Stadium behind the red, white, and blue was too much to pass up. Over 125,000 people in the stands were cheering and screaming, and felt like it was just for us. The Aussie fans were incredible. I really felt at home.

A few days later my parents and sister arrived. They took out a second mortgage to pay for their trip, but as they said, there was no way that they would miss their son/brother in the Olympic Games. Leading up to the race, the trainers worked really hard to get my piriformis better. When race day came I thought I was ready. There were 52 men on the start line, each wanting to perform their best. Every one of them had dreamed of winning a medal at the Olympic Games since they were kids. Now was our chance. The race started by walking 2km on the track, followed by 2km to get over to the 2km course where we would do 7 laps, and then walk 2km back to the stadium. My first 2km was in 8:01. I was on schedule. The next kilometer leaving the stadium, heading out through the tunnel and onto the road, was in 3:58. I felt great. The next kilometer was in 4:05. Still felt super, and we were finally onto the Olympic 2km course. Then disaster began to strike. The first time I went past the judge from the U.S., she showed me a caution paddle. It is rare for a judge to give "their" own country's athlete a caution, much less a red card. I was frustrated by this. In my opinion this was the case of an American official trying to show non-bias. One lap later, I was the first person in the race with a red card on the board. By 8km, I had my second red card on the board. One more and I would be disqualified. I did not work this hard, and suffer through difficult workouts every other day to get disqualified.

I began to slow and tried concentrating on my technique even more. I did not want to embarrass my family or my country. I knew one walker from a previous Olympics who was disqualified and to this day he was still kicking himself over it. I could not let that happen to me. The pain in my piriformis began to increase as my adrenalin began to subside. I went through 10km in 42:25. Still, not a bad time, if I could just hold it together. As the race wore on, I got into survival mode. I just kept putting one foot in front of the other with the absolute best technique I had. My times slowed dramatically and I just wished the pain and frustration would be over. I wanted to crawl into a hole and never be seen again. Finally, I entered the Olympic stadium. I finished the race in 40th place, beating just four lonely people, in a time of 1:30:32. This was not the way I wanted my Olympic experience to be.

Post Olympics

I walked away from my first Olympics $15,000 in debt and feeling utterly discouraged. I would not walk another step for two months. The U.S. Olympic Committee warned us multiple times about something they called Post-Olympic depression. The reason many athletes got this is because the Olympics were such a high for them, when they returned home they had trouble adapting to being a normal person again. I was determined not to let this happen to me and worked toward my next Olympic berth.

While it is a tale for another day, my second appearance in the Olympic Games was far more successful. I finished 20th with the fastest 20km American time at an Olympic Games, completing the course in 1:25:19, just a scant few seconds ahead of my teammate, training partner, and best friend Kevin Eastler.

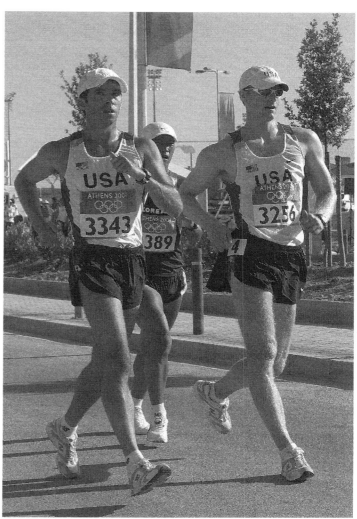

Tim Seaman and Kevin Eastler walking to Olympic success in 2004.

Appendix A: Pace Chart

km / Hour	Pace / km	Pace / mile	Pace / 400m
6	10:00	16:05	4:01
6.	9:13	14:51	3:42
7	8:34	13:47	3:26
7.5	8:00	12:52	3:13
8	7:30	12:04	3:01
8.5	7:03	11:21	2:50
9	6:40	10:43	2:41
9.5	6:18	10:09	2:32
10	6:00	9:39	2:24
10.5	5:42	9:11	2:16
11	5:27	8:46	2:10
11.5	5:13	8:23	2:05
12	5:00	8:02	2:00
12.5	4:48	7:43	1:56
13	4:36	7:25	1:51
13.5	4:26	7:09	1:47
14	4:17	6:53	1:42
14.5	4:08	6:39	1:39
15	4:00	6:24	1:36
15.5	3:52	6:14	1:33
16	3:45	6:00	1:30

Appendix B: Heart Rate Based Zone Calculations

Theoretical Max HR	Zone #1 HR (Min)	Zone #1 HR (Max)	Zone #2 HR (Min)	Zone #2 HR (Max)	Zone #3 HR (Min)	Zone #3 HR (Max)	Zone #4 HR (Min)	Zone #4 HR (Max)
220	154	165	167	187	189	198	200	209
215	151	161	163	183	185	194	196	204
210	147	158	160	179	181	189	191	200
205	144	154	156	174	176	185	187	195
200	140	150	152	170	172	180	182	190
195	137	146	148	166	168	176	177	185
190	133	143	144	162	163	171	173	181
185	130	139	141	157	159	167	168	176
180	126	135	137	153	155	162	164	171
175	123	131	133	149	151	158	159	166
170	119	128	129	145	146	153	155	162
165	116	124	125	140	142	149	150	157
160	112	120	122	136	138	144	146	152
155	109	116	118	132	133	140	141	147
150	105	113	114	128	129	135	137	143
145	102	109	110	123	125	131	132	138
140	98	105	106	119	120	126	127	133
135	95	101	103	115	116	122	123	128
130	91	98	99	111	112	117	118	124
125	88	94	95	106	108	113	114	119
120	84	90	91	102	103	108	109	114
115	81	86	87	98	99	104	105	109
110	77	83	84	94	95	99	100	105
105	74	79	80	89	90	95	96	100
100	70	75	76	85	86	90	91	95

Appendix C: Pace Based Zone Calculations

10 km Race	20 km Race	Zone 1		Zone 2		Zone 3		Zone 4	
		Upper	Lower	Upper	Lower	Upper	Lower	Upper	Lower
39:06	1:21:30	5:18	4:51	4:48	4:20	4:17	3:53	3:51	3:42
39:20	1:22:00	5:19	4:53	4:49	4:22	4:19	3:54	3:52	3:44
39:35	1:22:30	5:21	4:55	4:51	4:23	4:21	3:56	3:53	3:45
39:49	1:23:00	5:23	4:56	4:53	4:25	4:22	3:57	3:55	3:46
40:03	1:23:30	5:25	4:58	4:55	4:26	4:24	3:59	3:56	3:48
40:18	1:24:00	5:27	5:00	4:56	4:28	4:25	4:00	3:58	3:49
40:32	1:24:30	5:29	5:02	4:58	4:30	4:27	4:01	3:59	3:50
40:46	1:25:00	5:31	5:04	5:00	4:31	4:28	4:03	4:01	3:52
41:01	1:25:30	5:33	5:05	5:02	4:33	4:30	4:04	4:02	3:53
41:15	1:26:00	5:35	5:07	5:04	4:34	4:32	4:06	4:03	3:55
41:30	1:26:30	5:37	5:09	5:05	4:36	4:33	4:07	4:05	3:56
41:44	1:27:00	5:39	5:11	5:07	4:38	4:35	4:09	4:06	3:57
41:58	1:27:30	5:41	5:13	5:09	4:39	4:36	4:10	4:08	3:59
42:13	1:28:00	5:43	5:14	5:11	4:41	4:38	4:11	4:09	4:00
42:27	1:28:30	5:45	5:16	5:12	4:42	4:39	4:13	4:10	4:01
42:42	1:29:00	5:47	5:18	5:14	4:44	4:41	4:14	4:12	4:03
42:56	1:29:30	5:49	5:20	5:16	4:46	4:43	4:16	4:13	4:04
43:10	1:30:00	5:51	5:21	5:18	4:47	4:44	4:17	4:15	4:05
43:25	1:30:30	5:53	5:23	5:19	4:49	4:46	4:19	4:16	4:07
43:39	1:31:00	5:55	5:25	5:21	4:50	4:47	4:20	4:18	4:08
43:54	1:31:30	5:56	5:27	5:23	4:52	4:49	4:21	4:19	4:10
44:08	1:32:00	5:58	5:29	5:25	4:54	4:51	4:23	4:20	4:11
44:22	1:32:30	6:00	5:30	5:26	4:55	4:52	4:24	4:22	4:12
44:37	1:33:00	6:02	5:32	5:28	4:57	4:54	4:26	4:23	4:14
44:51	1:33:30	6:04	5:34	5:30	4:58	4:55	4:27	4:25	4:15
45:06	1:34:00	6:06	5:36	5:32	5:00	4:57	4:29	4:26	4:16
45:20	1:34:30	6:08	5:38	5:34	5:02	4:58	4:30	4:27	4:18
45:34	1:35:00	6:10	5:39	5:35	5:03	5:00	4:31	4:29	4:19
45:49	1:35:30	6:12	5:41	5:37	5:05	5:02	4:33	4:30	4:20
46:03	1:36:00	6:14	5:43	5:39	5:06	5:03	4:34	4:32	4:22
46:17	1:36:30	6:16	5:45	5:41	5:08	5:05	4:36	4:33	4:23
46:32	1:37:00	6:18	5:46	5:42	5:10	5:06	4:37	4:35	4:25
46:46	1:37:30	6:20	5:48	5:44	5:11	5:08	4:39	4:36	4:26
47:01	1:38:00	6:22	5:50	5:46	5:13	5:09	4:40	4:37	4:27

10 km Race	20 km Race	Zone 1		Zone 2		Zone 3		Zone 4	
		Upper	Lower	Upper	Lower	Upper	Lower	Upper	Lower
47:15	1:38:30	6:24	5:52	5:48	5:14	5:11	4:41	4:39	4:29
47:29	1:39:00	6:26	5:54	5:49	5:16	5:13	4:43	4:40	4:30
47:44	1:39:30	6:28	5:55	5:51	5:18	5:14	4:44	4:42	4:31
47:58	1:40:00	6:30	5:57	5:53	5:19	5:16	4:46	4:43	4:33
48:13	1:40:30	6:32	5:59	5:55	5:21	5:17	4:47	4:44	4:34
48:27	1:41:00	6:34	6:01	5:56	5:22	5:19	4:49	4:46	4:35
48:41	1:41:30	6:35	6:03	5:58	5:24	5:21	4:50	4:47	4:37
48:56	1:42:00	6:37	6:04	6:00	5:26	5:22	4:51	4:49	4:38
49:10	1:42:30	6:39	6:06	6:02	5:27	5:24	4:53	4:50	4:40
49:25	1:43:00	6:41	6:08	6:04	5:29	5:25	4:54	4:52	4:41
49:39	1:43:30	6:43	6:10	6:05	5:30	5:27	4:56	4:53	4:42
49:53	1:44:00	6:45	6:11	6:07	5:32	5:28	4:57	4:54	4:44
50:08	1:44:30	6:47	6:13	6:09	5:34	5:30	4:59	4:56	4:45
50:22	1:45:00	6:49	6:15	6:11	5:35	5:32	5:00	4:57	4:46
50:37	1:45:30	6:51	6:17	6:12	5:37	5:33	5:01	4:59	4:48
50:51	1:46:00	6:53	6:19	6:14	5:38	5:35	5:03	5:00	4:49
51:05	1:46:30	6:55	6:20	6:16	5:40	5:36	5:04	5:01	4:50
51:20	1:47:00	6:57	6:22	6:18	5:41	5:38	5:06	5:03	4:52
51:34	1:47:30	6:59	6:24	6:19	5:43	5:39	5:07	5:04	4:53
51:48	1:48:00	7:01	6:26	6:21	5:45	5:41	5:09	5:06	4:55
52:03	1:48:30	7:03	6:28	6:23	5:46	5:43	5:10	5:07	4:56
52:17	1:49:00	7:05	6:29	6:25	5:48	5:44	5:11	5:08	4:57
52:32	1:49:30	7:07	6:31	6:26	5:49	5:46	5:13	5:10	4:59
52:46	1:50:00	7:09	6:33	6:28	5:51	5:47	5:14	5:11	5:00
53:00	1:50:30	7:11	6:35	6:30	5:53	5:49	5:16	5:13	5:01
53:15	1:51:00	7:12	6:36	6:32	5:54	5:51	5:17	5:14	5:03
53:29	1:51:30	7:14	6:38	6:34	5:56	5:52	5:19	5:16	5:04
53:44	1:52:00	7:16	6:40	6:35	5:57	5:54	5:20	5:17	5:05
53:58	1:52:30	7:18	6:42	6:37	5:59	5:55	5:21	5:18	5:07
54:12	1:53:00	7:20	6:44	6:39	6:01	5:57	5:23	5:20	5:08
54:27	1:53:30	7:22	6:45	6:41	6:02	5:58	5:24	5:21	5:10
54:41	1:54:00	7:24	6:47	6:42	6:04	6:00	5:26	5:23	5:11
54:56	1:54:30	7:26	6:49	6:44	6:05	6:02	5:27	5:24	5:12
55:10	1:55:00	7:28	6:51	6:46	6:07	6:03	5:29	5:25	5:14
55:24	1:55:30	7:30	6:53	6:48	6:09	6:05	5:30	5:27	5:15
55:39	1:56:00	7:32	6:54	6:49	6:10	6:06	5:31	5:28	5:16
55:53	1:56:30	7:34	6:56	6:51	6:12	6:08	5:33	5:30	5:18

10 km Race	20 km Race	Zone 1		Zone 2		Zone 3		Zone 4	
		Upper	Lower	Upper	Lower	Upper	Lower	Upper	Lower
56:08	1:57:00	7:36	6:58	6:53	6:13	6:09	5:34	5:31	5:19
56:22	1:57:30	7:38	6:60	6:55	6:15	6:11	5:36	5:33	5:20
56:36	1:58:00	7:40	7:01	6:56	6:17	6:13	5:37	5:34	5:22
56:51	1:58:30	7:42	7:03	6:58	6:18	6:14	5:39	5:35	5:23
57:05	1:59:00	7:44	7:05	7:00	6:20	6:16	5:40	5:37	5:25
57:19	1:59:30	7:46	7:07	7:02	6:21	6:17	5:41	5:38	5:26
57:34	2:00:00	7:48	7:09	7:04	6:23	6:19	5:43	5:40	5:27
57:48	2:00:30	7:49	7:10	7:05	6:25	6:21	5:44	5:41	5:29
58:03	2:01:00	7:51	7:12	7:07	6:26	6:22	5:46	5:42	5:30
58:17	2:01:30	7:53	7:14	7:09	6:28	6:24	5:47	5:44	5:31
58:31	2:02:00	7:55	7:16	7:11	6:29	6:25	5:49	5:45	5:33
58:46	2:02:30	7:57	7:18	7:12	6:31	6:27	5:50	5:47	5:34
59:00	2:03:00	7:59	7:19	7:14	6:33	6:28	5:51	5:48	5:35
59:15	2:03:30	8:01	7:21	7:16	6:34	6:30	5:53	5:50	5:37
59:29	2:04:00	8:03	7:23	7:18	6:36	6:32	5:54	5:51	5:38
59:43	2:04:30	8:05	7:25	7:19	6:37	6:33	5:56	5:52	5:40
59:58	2:05:00	8:07	7:26	7:21	6:39	6:35	5:57	5:54	5:41
60:12	2:05:30	8:09	7:28	7:23	6:41	6:36	5:59	5:55	5:42
60:27	2:06:00	8:11	7:30	7:25	6:42	6:38	6:00	5:57	5:44
60:41	2:06:30	8:13	7:32	7:26	6:44	6:39	6:01	5:58	5:45
60:55	2:07:00	8:15	7:34	7:28	6:45	6:41	6:03	5:59	5:46
61:10	2:07:30	8:17	7:35	7:30	6:47	6:43	6:04	6:01	5:48
61:24	2:08:00	8:19	7:37	7:32	6:49	6:44	6:06	6:02	5:49
61:39	2:08:30	8:21	7:39	7:34	6:50	6:46	6:07	6:04	5:50
61:53	2:09:00	8:23	7:41	7:35	6:52	6:47	6:09	6:05	5:52
62:07	2:09:30	8:25	7:43	7:37	6:53	6:49	6:10	6:07	5:53
62:22	2:10:00	8:26	7:44	7:39	6:55	6:51	6:11	6:08	5:55
62:36	2:10:30	8:28	7:46	7:41	6:56	6:52	6:13	6:09	5:56
62:50	2:11:00	8:30	7:48	7:42	6:58	6:54	6:14	6:11	5:57
63:05	2:11:30	8:32	7:50	7:44	6:60	6:55	6:16	6:12	5:59
63:19	2:12:00	8:34	7:51	7:46	7:01	6:57	6:17	6:14	6:00
63:34	2:12:30	8:36	7:53	7:48	7:03	6:58	6:19	6:15	6:01
63:48	2:13:00	8:38	7:55	7:49	7:04	7:00	6:20	6:16	6:03
64:02	2:13:30	8:40	7:57	7:51	7:06	7:02	6:21	6:18	6:04
64:17	2:14:00	8:42	7:59	7:53	7:08	7:03	6:23	6:19	6:05
64:31	2:14:30	8:44	8:00	7:55	7:09	7:05	6:24	6:21	6:07
64:46	2:15:00	8:46	8:02	7:56	7:11	7:06	6:26	6:22	6:08

10 km Race	20 km Race	Zone 1		Zone 2		Zone 3		Zone 4	
		Upper	Lower	Upper	Lower	Upper	Lower	Upper	Lower
65:00	2:15:30	8:48	8:04	7:58	7:12	7:08	6:27	6:23	6:10
65:14	2:16:00	8:50	8:06	8:00	7:14	7:09	6:29	6:25	6:11
65:29	2:16:30	8:52	8:08	8:02	7:16	7:11	6:30	6:26	6:12
65:43	2:17:00	8:54	8:09	8:04	7:17	7:13	6:31	6:28	6:14
65:58	2:17:30	8:56	8:11	8:05	7:19	7:14	6:33	6:29	6:15
66:12	2:18:00	8:58	8:13	8:07	7:20	7:16	6:34	6:31	6:16
66:26	2:18:30	8:60	8:15	8:09	7:22	7:17	6:36	6:32	6:18
66:41	2:19:00	9:02	8:16	8:11	7:24	7:19	6:37	6:33	6:19
66:55	2:19:30	9:04	8:18	8:12	7:25	7:21	6:39	6:35	6:20
67:10	2:20:00	9:05	8:20	8:14	7:27	7:22	6:40	6:36	6:22
67:24	2:20:30	9:07	8:22	8:16	7:28	7:24	6:41	6:38	6:23
67:38	2:21:00	9:09	8:24	8:18	7:30	7:25	6:43	6:39	6:25
67:53	2:21:30	9:11	8:25	8:19	7:32	7:27	6:44	6:40	6:26
68:07	2:22:00	9:13	8:27	8:21	7:33	7:28	6:46	6:42	6:27
68:21	2:22:30	9:15	8:29	8:23	7:35	7:30	6:47	6:43	6:29
68:36	2:23:00	9:17	8:31	8:25	7:36	7:32	6:49	6:45	6:30
68:50	2:23:30	9:19	8:33	8:26	7:38	7:33	6:50	6:46	6:31
69:05	2:24:00	9:21	8:34	8:28	7:40	7:35	6:51	6:48	6:33
69:19	2:24:30	9:23	8:36	8:30	7:41	7:36	6:53	6:49	6:34
69:33	2:25:00	9:25	8:38	8:32	7:43	7:38	6:54	6:50	6:35
69:48	2:25:30	9:27	8:40	8:34	7:44	7:39	6:56	6:52	6:37
70:02	2:26:00	9:29	8:41	8:35	7:46	7:41	6:57	6:53	6:38
70:17	2:26:30	9:31	8:43	8:37	7:48	7:43	6:59	6:55	6:40
70:31	2:27:00	9:33	8:45	8:39	7:49	7:44	7:00	6:56	6:41
70:45	2:27:30	9:35	8:47	8:41	7:51	7:46	7:01	6:57	6:42
70:60	2:28:00	9:37	8:49	8:42	7:52	7:47	7:03	6:59	6:44
71:14	2:28:30	9:39	8:50	8:44	7:54	7:49	7:04	7:00	6:45
71:29	2:29:00	9:41	8:52	8:46	7:56	7:51	7:06	7:02	6:46
71:43	2:29:30	9:42	8:54	8:48	7:57	7:52	7:07	7:03	6:48
71:57	2:30:00	9:44	8:56	8:49	7:59	7:54	7:09	7:05	6:49

Appendix D: Altitude Training Locations

The following is a list of places that are ideal, or close to ideal, for altitude training camps:

Flagstaff, AZ - By far my most favorite place to train at altitude. With an altitude of around 7,000 feet (2,100m), pretty good weather almost year round, and with some higher peaks for hiking just outside the city limits, Flagstaff offers athletes a great over-all climate for training. We typically rent a condo or house with room for three to six athletes in each unit. This keeps the costs manageable. For those athletes in the U.S., Flagstaff is easy to get to via car or plane through Phoenix or directly into Flagstaff. If you are going to train here, though, we recommend you have a car so you can get around to the different training sites.

St. Moritz, Switzerland -   While I have personally never trained there, my Team Plaetzer teammates have used this 1,856m high oasis every summer before their big championship races. The views alone make it priceless. Typically they rent a condo and are able to train on either the track or the 4km loop around the airport. For endurance athletes, though, it would be best to utilize this location in the summer time, since the snow can be a deterrent during the winter months.

Font Romeu, France - A favorite with the Spanish National Team for the past 30 years, athletes like World Champions Valenti Masana, Jose Marin and Jesus Garcia have trained there for three to four weeks at a time to prepare for their major championships. Since it is just a short two-hour drive from Barcelona it is especially convenient. The Centre National d'Entrainement en Altitude (CNEA) is located in the Pyrenees on a plateau of 1850 meters. For more information go to www.cnea-fontromeu.com

Colorado Springs, Colorado - This 6,000-foot (1,840m) high city is the home of the U.S. Olympic Training Center and is in the shadow of Pikes Peak. With the snow capped mountains in the background, this city has really taken on the Olympic spirit full force. While the weather can get tricky in the winter, this is a very good location with tons of trails and paths to train on. If you are good enough to get access to the Olympic Training Center, take the opportunity, because the Sports Science staff is top notch.

Mexico City, Mexico - In 1968 when Mexico surprised the world with a bronze medal in the 20km walk, the race walking community took notice of the Centro Deportivo Olympico Mexicano (CDOM) and has been intrigued ever since. There are sometimes up to 50 athletes coached by 6 different coaches. While this could be an ideal place to train, it has drawbacks. The pollution is so bad that training must start at 6 am before the pollution gets into the "danger" level. Currently I would not recommend going there to train because if the pollution doesn't get you, the muggers and kidnappers just might.

ADDITIONAL PUBLICATIONS BY WALKING PROMOTIONS

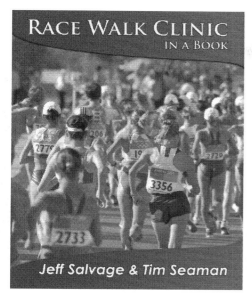

America's premier team of clinicians Jeff Salvage and Tim Seaman's *Race Walk Clinic — in a Book* beautifully illustrates textbook techniques while it catalogs typical mistakes race walkers make that can rob them of a legal race and speed. It explains why these problems exist and prescribes critical solutions to correct them. If you are ready to improve your race walking style and step up to the next level, then pick up *Race Walk Clinic - in a Book* today. Our approach in *Race Walk Clinic — in a Book* is to pick up where other training materials leave off. We start by grounding our discussion with a review of correct race walking technique, but do not focus on the many aspects of technique that you can do incorrectly. We then divide race walking technique problems into broad categories, starting with issues of legality and then separating technique issues into categories such as hip, leg, arm, and posture problems. For each category we illustrate the problem with photographs of either elite race walkers or (for beginner problems) staged images. We then offer remediation in two forms: exercises, drills and stretches to improve your style; and mental cues to guide your focus while race walking. Within the educational material presented, we've interspersed "Tales from the Track," a unique collection of stories in which great race walkers from the U.S. and around the world retell some of their most memorable experiences.

Order from www.racewalk.com or www.racewalkclinic.com for $23.95 + S & H

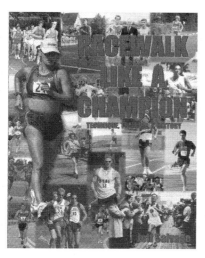

Printed with 8 1/2 x 11 full-color pages, *Race Walk Like a Champion* is the single best compilation of information on the technique, training, and history of race walking. It combines approximately 400 photographs with charts and diagrams to explain every detail of race walking. *Race Walk Like a Champion* starts with a thorough explanation of how to select race walking shoes and warm-up; it then describes every aspect of race walking technique, judging, and training philosophy in extensive detail. Other chapters include stretching, racing, strength training, mental preparation, injury treatment, and nutrition. *Race Walk Like a Champion* also includes a comprehensive chapter on the history of American race walking. Each era of walking is described with an introduction and biographies of that period's greats.

Order from www.racewalk.com for $23.95 + S & H

ADDITIONAL PUBLICATIONS BY WALKING PROMOTIONS

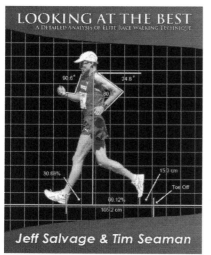

Looking at the Best, A Detailed Analysis of Elite Race Walking Technique takes the discussion of race walking locomotion further than ever before. By combining high resolution - high speed photography with computer software and detailed measurements, we paint an image of exactly how the best race walkers in the world stride forward at speeds approaching 10 mph (16 kph). Instead of theorizing the body motions comprising ideal race walking technique, we analyze the race walkers from elite race walk competitions featuring the very best race walkers in the world.

Under race conditions (primarily at the 12th World Championships in Berlin), we see the good, bad and ugly with regard to technique. By using real race photographs we take the discussion out of the proverbial laboratory and examine how race walkers do what we want to do, race fast.

Order from www.racewalk.com for $27.95 + S & H

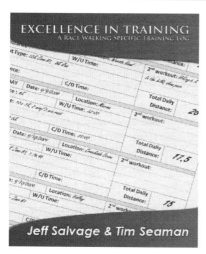

We all know we should keep a training log. Some of us do, and others don't get beyond the new season's resolution to keep better track of our workouts. Those keeping track, often do so inconsistently. Now let America's premier team of clinicians Jeff Salvage and Tim Seaman help you record information vital to your race walking progress in *Excellence in Training – A Race Walking Specific Training Log*.

Excellence in Training has space for 52 weeks of 7 days a week training. Each day has space for the date, location of the workout, warm-up distance, warm-up pace, workout type, cool down distance, cool down time, additional space for splits or notes about the workout, total daily distance, and room for a second workout.

Order from www.racewalk.com or www.racewalkclinic.com $19.95 for 1 copy or $30.00 for 2 copies + S&H

ADDITIONAL PUBLICATIONS BY WALKING PROMOTIONS

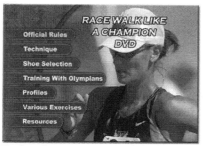

The *Race Walk Like a Champion* companion DVD/CD brings the descriptions from the book to life while explaining all aspects of race walking in DVD-quality video. However, the benefits of the DVD format do not end there; the interactivity makes it a coach in a box. Its friendly menus allow you to watch exactly the section you wish, over and over, with no rewinding! Have a technique problem? Just drill down through the interactive menus and your ever-present coach is there to assist.

Order from www.racewalk.com for $49.95 + S&H

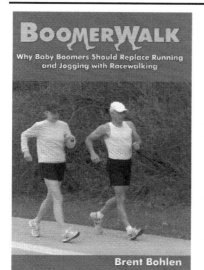

If you are reading this page, you clearly are already interested in race walking and have a strong knowledge of the sport. How about inspiring one of the 75 million baby boomers who need to learn about our great sport? **BoomerWalk** is written to inspire a wide range of people to become race walkers. It is a great summary of basic technique that motivates readers to get off the couch and start race walking. Author Brent Bohlen relates his experience in discovering the sport of race walking at a time in his life when his aging knees no longer could take the pounding of his four-decade love of basketball. Race walking provided him the cardiovascular fitness he needed, the competition he wanted, and the kindness his knees demanded. Once he convinces you to take up race walking, whether for fitness or for competition, Bohlen provides the basics of race walking technique to get you off on the right foot. You can begin race walking right away with no special equipment.

Order from www.BoomerWalk.com, www.racewalk.com, or www.amazon.com for $15.95 + S&H.

Please visit WWW.RACEWALK.COM for the latest information about race walking and don't forget to join our electronic newsletter by signing up on our homepage.

ATTEND A CLINIC OF EXCELLENCE

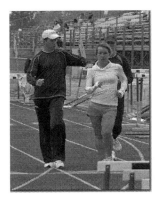

Books and DVDs are great ways to expand your knowledge of race walking, but nothing helps more than an in person experience with a coach. If you are a beginner wishing to learn the basics or a seasoned race walker looking to improve your technique and training program, then you are ready to be an excellent race walker. Attend a *Clinic of Excellence* by two-time Olympian Tim Seaman and founder of www.racewalk.com Jeff Salvage. Tim's experience as one of America's most dominant 20K walkers for the past two decades combined with Jeff's vast experience of coaching, educating, and promoting race walking come together in a weekend clinic that features individualized attention, group lectures, and high tech know how that will leave you walking more quickly, more legally, and more powerfully than before.

Featuring not one but two qualified instructors allows the clinics to focus on beginners and advanced walkers simultaneously. All attendees will experience hands on coaching, in addition to the many well prepared lectures covering technique, training philosophy, nutrition, injuries, and strength work. Jeff's unparalleled photographs of the World's best walkers along with Tim's critique of their style provides unique insight into the upper echelon of race walking. While many walkers need the detailed PowerPoint presentation on technique, others who have attended clinics in the past can opt for additional hands on experience with Tim. All participants will not only receive individualized attention and feedback, but will also receive an electronic version of their images with the critiques sketched overtop. In addition, we just added the ability for attendees to take home video footage of their newly learned race walking style.

Tim Seaman has race walked since 1988 and quickly became one of America's premier race walkers. He broke his first Jr. Record in 1990 and was a member of the 2000 and 2004 Olympic team. Tim is second on the all time American list of national titles and currently holds 10 American records. In addition to training and working, Tim has coached some of America's top National Team women as well as many of the best and brightest upcoming stars from the South Texas Walking Club and from around the country.

Jeff Salvage started race walking in 1984 and had a brief, but successful, career competing nationally and internationally as a competitor before turning to coaching and educating. He is the founder of www.racewalk.com and author of "Walk Like an Athlete" and "Race Walk Like a Champion" as well as their corresponding videos and DVDs. Jeff has coached walkers at all levels from beginning fitness walkers, marathoners, elite juniors, and international competitors.

ARE YOU READY TO BE EXCELLENT? Then check out www.racewalkclinic.com for a schedule of our upcoming clinics.

Made in the USA
Lexington, KY
23 October 2013